Estrogen Dominance

Hormonal Imbalance
of the 21st Century

Michael Lam, M.D., M.P.H.
Dorine Lam, R.D., M.S., M.P.H.

Estrogen Dominance: Hormonal Imbalance of the 21st Century
by Michael Lam, M.D., M.P.H. and Dorine Lam, R.D., M.S., M.P.H.

© Copyright 2008-2012 by Michael Lam, M.D.

Published in the United States by:

Adrenal Institute Press, Loma Linda, CA 92354
www.AdrenalInstitute.org

Cover and Interior Design: Nick Zelinger, NZ Graphics
Editing: John Maling (Editing By John), Virginia McCullough
Book Shepherding: Judith Briles

ISBN (paperback): 978-1-937930-11-0
ISBN (ebook): 978-1-937930-12-7
Library of Congress Control Number: 2012905805

Estrogen Dominance: Hormonal Imbalance of the 21st Century / Michael Lam, Dorine Lam. Second edition, 2012

10 9 8 7 6 5 4 3 2 1

1. Health   2. Adrenal glands—Disease.   3. Fatigue   4. Stress (Physiology)   5. Neuroendocrine

Second Edition

Printed in the United States of America

Contents

Author's Note

Many of the disorders encountered today were unknown and unheard of a mere century ago. Technology and the multitude of new chemicals and other agents of modernization cause a host of illnesses and health problems.

Chief among these silent killers is hormone estrogen when present in excess amounts. Sometimes the danger comes in the guise of useful household products that we buy off the shelf that have chemical structures akin to those of estrogen. Hormone-laced beef and poultry, pesticides, car pollutants and the leftover estrogen from hormone replacement therapy (HRT) are all culprits

You may not have known it but you are bathing in a sea of estrogen and estrogen-like compounds created by our industrial world over the past 100 years.

The hormonal imbalance caused by excessive estrogen has brought us a myriad of illnesses including premenstrual syndrome (PMS), premenopausal syndrome, uterine fibroids, breast cysts, endometriosis, and breast cancer. Many women develop the entire series. The list is not exhaustive and these illnesses are not mutually exclusive. Many women develop the entire series—the root cause is the same.

It's time to clear up the misinformation and ignorance. *Estrogen Dominance* will be your guide.

Dr. Lam

Note: This book is part of Dr. Lam's Adrenal Recovery Series. This book provides a more in-depth look into Estrogen Dominance. Sections of this book can be found in *Adrenal Fatigue Syndrome: Reclaim Your Energy and Vitality with Clinically Proven Natural Programs.*

Introduction

It is no longer surprising news that many of the disorders we encounter today were unknown and unheard of a mere century ago. Certainly, we can count many technological advances in the 20th century that the world can be very proud of. But these achievements have come at a very high price in terms of public health. It has become more and more clear that the multitude of new chemicals and other agents of modernization are causing a host of illnesses and health problems. Some of these are so toxic that they have been banned or are much controlled in their use. Others are more insidious, undermining our health, unnoticed over years before their effects are noticed.

Chief among these silent killers is the hormone estrogen when present in excess amount. The situation has been worsened because of the short-term benefits from employing the hormone. Sometimes the danger comes in the guise of useful household products that we buy off the shelf. They have chemical structures akin to those of estrogen. You get them in hormone-laced beef and poultry, pesticides, car pollutants and the leftover estrogen from hormone replacement therapy (HRT). You may not have known it but you are bathing in a sea of estrogen and estrogen-like compounds created by our industrial world over the past 100 years.

The hormonal imbalance caused by excessive estrogen has brought us a myriad of illnesses including premenstrual syndrome (PMS), premenopausal syndrome, uterine fibroids, breast cysts, endometriosis, and breast cancer. Many women develop the entire series. The list is not exhaustive and these illnesses are not mutually exclusive. They are manifestations of the same underlying problem—estrogen dominance—a condition in which estrogen overwhelms the other hormones that normally work in a harmonious cycle with it. When and in which part of the body it flares up may be different from one patient to another but the root cause is the same.

Misinformation and ignorance since the mid 1960s is all to blame. The good news is that the excess estrogen can be neutralized. Natural medicine deploying natural hormones and nutritional supplements can help. This book is a resource that details the syndromes caused and remedies available to sufferers of hormonal imbalances. It is written for every woman wanting to reverse the odds of developing these diseases of the modern world. There are simple, life-saving solutions and advice, whether you are showing early signs of estrogen dominance like PMS or menopausal problems, or more advanced deterioration such as breast cancer. You just cannot afford not to know. The consequence of ignorance can kill you!

Michael Lam M.D. M.P.H.

Part 1
THE PROBLEM

Chapter 1

Jane's Story—A Woman's Struggle with Estrogen Dominance

Little Jane stood by her mother's grave sobbing uncontrollably. They had just buried her mother, a victim of the dreaded breast cancer. As she placed some flowers on the grave, Jane could not understand why her mother had been taken away from her. At the tender age of ten, Jane could not fully comprehend the meaning of cancer and death.

After her mother passed away, she was raised by the rest of her family and managed to lead a seemingly normal and healthy childhood. At the age of 13, Jane entered puberty and had her first menstrual period. Her body developed and blossomed, she filled out and she became more conscious of her appearance. By the time she reached 18 years of age, she had a full, womanly figure. She was growing very attractive and had many boyfriends.

As A Teenager

Jane took birth control pills during the last two years of her high school. After she entered college, she took less of it as she became sexually less active. Due to her increased workload in college, she found less time for socializing. Likewise, Jane did not devote much time to exercise, although she did go to the college gym for a simple workout with her girlfriends at least once a month. Her appetite was good and she began to put on a little weight because of her new craving for sweets like chocolate, donuts and ice cream. But she was not obese by any means.

Maturing Into an Adult

Upon graduation, Jane found a job as an advertising executive in a large corporation in the city. To save commuting time, she moved from the suburb into the city. She bought a charming house near her workplace. A few years later, at the age of 25, she met and eventually married her husband. She was a good home maker and kept their home tidy and neat using everyday detergents and other household chemicals. They maintained a garden and, to keep the flowers free of insects and pests, they applied pesticides regularly.

As she got caught up in her work, Jane became more and more of a workaholic. She worked an average of 12 hours a day. Her bosses recognized her talents and efforts and promoted her to middle management a few years later. Jane was ecstatic and felt a sense of achievement. She was only in her thirties and she already had a staff of 20 people under her. Her personal office had a panoramic view of the city.

Jane's work was mainly sedentary. She had plenty of meetings to attend, both locally and overseas. Her job responsibilities included meeting important clients and business development as well as developing new strategic plans for her company. She tried to go to the gym weekly despite the many chores she had to attend to at work and at home.

Jane was grateful that despite her stressful life at the office, her health was good. Her hormonal history was actually quite mundane. When she was in her teens, her periods were regular and normal. It was only after her marriage that she would miss a period here and there, especially when she was under severe stress at work.

In the office, Jane drank one to two cups of coffee a day to keep herself awake and alert. She was told that coffee was not good for her and, over the years, reduced her intake replacing it with black tea. When she traveled, she would skip her regular exercise program as she simply could not afford the time. Gradually, she gained more weight, especially in the waistline, due to the lavish meals, rich in meat and alcohol, in the course of entertaining clients.

Being a career woman, Jane believed that she had managed her life well enough. Despite her long working hours, she still managed to get about five to six hours of sleep a night and at least one weekend off a month to be with her family. Significantly, outside her bedroom window there was a street lamp which served as her nightlight when the blinds were not drawn closed. Therefore, she usually did not sleep in total darkness.

After five years of marriage, she gave birth to her first child at the age of 31. Following the birth, Jane's menstrual period started to become irregular. She began to notice the onset of slight headaches, bloating, and cramps, and felt irritable before and during midcycle in her period. She ignored these symptoms as they did not really hurt her too much and continued to work just as hard. On days when she was unable to cope with the symptoms, she would resort to taking an aspirin or perhaps a few hours of sleep to recuperate.

Once, she visited her family doctor to find out if anything was amiss. He assured her that these were normal premenstrual symptoms. As the symptoms did not affect her greatly, he just told her to learn to live with them.

At age 33 Jane gave birth to her second child, a daughter. She decided that two was enough. Her doctor suggested a simple procedure called tubal ligation where the fallopian tubes are tied. This was the best means of birth control, according to her doctors. She had it done and it was uneventful. With the passage of time, her PMS got progressively worse. Whenever she was under stress, she would also miss a period now and again. A strong woman, she was able to continue her demanding work schedule despite the attacks. Once or twice she needed time off to tide her over the PMS. Hyper-pigmentation began to affect her face whenever she had her periods.

Approaching Menopause

Ten years down the road, as she continued to rise up the corporate ladder, her workload became even more punishing. While she tried to reduce her coffee intake and switch to tea, her overall consumption of caffeine had not reduced. She needed the stimulant to sustain her energy level. Exercise was seldom on her agenda. Fatty food was the norm as her entertainment schedule intensified the higher she rose in the corporation.

Jane started to experience slight depression and inexplicable anxiety. She became very conscious of her weight problem and enrolled herself in diet classes and even took diet pills. Despite these sporadic efforts, she failed to lose any weight. Her appetite grew and she felt hungry all the time. This happened more often after a heavy meal high in carbohydrates. As age was catching up with her, she often felt fatigued or sleepy, especially after eating.

One day, at a regular checkup, the doctor told her that her blood cholesterol level was slightly on the high side. As her fasting blood sugar was fine, he did not prescribe her any medication. He just told her to avoid stress and exercise more often.

Jane's weight continued to creep up. She began to notice more acne and coarse hair on her face. After she celebrated her 40th birthday, her menstrual flow became heavier and her premenstrual headaches and cramps became more severe.

Two years later, in an ultrasound scan of her uterus as part of her annual gynecological examination, her doctor found a fibroid, a ball of fibrous tissue measuring about two inches in diameter. She was only 42 years old. The doctor said that the tumor was benign and she should just leave it alone unless she had heavy bleeding. Poor Jane was scared to death. She sought comfort from many of her good friends with the same problems and found that the advice given by her doctor appeared to be quite standard and sound.

By the time she was 48, the fibroid was causing her to bleed heavily during her periods. As it began to press on her bladder, she had problems urinating. Jane underwent another ultrasound scan. This time, the doctor said that her fibroid had grown to about five inches in diameter and advised her to remove her uterus. Her ovaries were also to be removed. Her doctor said that as she was already approaching menopause, it did not matter whether she had her ovaries or not. Jane felt devastated but complied with her doctor's advice just the same.

After the surgery, she had her menopause right away with symptoms such as hot flashes. Her doctor started her on estrogen replacement therapy (ERT) to ease her symptoms. She was prescribed synthetic estrogen in a drug called Premarin®. He assured her that all would be well and that this ERT would protect her heart and prevent osteoporosis as well.

Much to her relief, Jane's hot flashes did improve with the synthetic estrogen. She remained on this drug faithfully even though she suffered the side effects of fatigue and bloating. As the years went by, her libido started to wane and depression began to beset her again. She started experiencing vaginal dryness and incontinence. Her skin became dry and she had more wrinkles on her face. These did nothing for her shriveling self-esteem and well-being. She related all these to the doctor but, once again, he assured her that these symptoms were very normal and that they were all part of the aging process. There was nothing much he could offer. He told Jane to adjust her expectations and accept the symptoms.

Jane accepted her doctor's analysis. After all, who would know better than her own doctor who had been treating her for so many years.

Jane tried to get on with her life and think positively. She assured herself that she did not have to worry about cancer, heart attack and osteoporosis as her uterus and ovaries had been removed. She was glad that she would definitely have no chances of getting cancer of the uterus or ovaries now.

Into Her Fifties

On a cold and frosty winter morning, Jane felt a lump in her left breast while she was bathing. She was mortified. Her husband rushed her to the hospital. There, she underwent a complete examination again. A biopsy confirmed her worst fears. The growth was a malignant tumor. Jane screamed. She had breast cancer! Her nightmares were coming true! And she was only 54.

The doctor suggested radical surgery—meaning the removal of the breast—and possibly chemotherapy after that. Jane was in a state of shock. She had been a perfect patient following everything the doctor recommended. How could this be happening to her? Her doctor did not give her a good explanation. He said these things were all part of life. She just had to learn to accept her cancer.

Jane and her family were told that immediate surgery was necessary to prevent further spread of the cancer. She was devastated but had no choice. So she underwent mastectomy followed by chemotherapy.

Looking Back a Little Too Late

Resting in the hospital after the surgery, Jane had much quiet time to reflect. She made up her mind to understand her own medical history. After her discharge from hospital, she surfed the Internet, talked to her friends and many naturally-oriented healthcare professionals, trying to piece together the facts of what really happened to her body. To her surprise, she discovered that her medical history was common to many women around her age. She realized that there are alternative solutions to her problems that her doctor was not aware of. She wished that her doctor had owned up to her earlier. She would definitely have looked at other options.

Jane's story is very real indeed. There are millions of women sharing this tragic background around the world; classic cases of repeated history.

Summary

In summary, Jane had been bathing in a sea of estrogen for 40 years without knowing it. Her body had been crying out for her to take notice, but she did not hear it. Finally, the body simply surrendered and Jane was stricken with cancer. Jane had it coming, if only she had known more about estrogen dominance. You may not see where Jane got her exogenous estrogen, but it was there, even though, like you, she did not realize it. We shall look into the details later. First, we need to have a basic understanding of how hormones work in our body.

Chapter 2

Hormones Acting in Concert

Before we can fully understand Jane's medical history, the alternative treatments open to her, and the current trends in managing sustainable good health and well-being, we need to comprehend the underlying processes in our body chemistry. It is important to appreciate what a beautiful system our body is. Pause for a moment to consider the many wonderful things we can do every day that we take for granted. All these complex tasks require a very sophisticated system of regulation and coordination.

One of the key regulatory systems in the body is the hormonal system. Hormones are very powerful chemicals that profoundly control and affect our body. Not surprisingly, they work in concert to maintain our health in an optimal state. These chemicals are produced in various glands and organs of the body, travel by way of the blood stream and effect certain actions in other glands and organs. There are hundreds of hormones in the body, all of which are important and serve interrelated and critical functions. Some hormones act to control other hormones, while others serve as precursors of another set of other hormones. We simply cannot survive without the proper functioning of the hormonal system. This is especially significant in the female due to its regulatory effect on the menstrual cycle.

These chemicals are secreted by glands which are collectively referred to as our endocrine system.

The Endocrine System

The endocrine system is made up of eight different glands located strategically throughout the body. They are the:

- Ovaries in women (in men, the testes)
- Adrenals
- Pancreas
- Thyroid
- Parathyroid
- Pineal
- Pituitary
- Hypothalamus (which is also part of the nervous system)

Together, the body's hormones regulate every aspect of life including reproduction; growth and development; the conversion of nutrients into energy in our body's cells (cellular metabolism); electrolytes and water balance; and the mobilization of body defenses against any microbes or chemicals that threaten our body. For our purpose, we will concentrate on the hormones related to the reproductive system as it is there that hormonal imbalance can cause real havoc in the body.

The Reproductive System

The control center of the female hormonal system lies in the hypothalamus. Here, a chemical called gonadotropin-releasing hormone (GnRH) is released. GnRH which signals the pituitary gland to secrete the follicle-stimulating hormone (FSH) and luteinizing Hormone (LH). FSH in turn travels to and stimulates the ovaries to secrete estrogen and other hormones that stimulate development of the breast, uterine and ovarian tissues and regulate the female reproductive system. Interestingly, the reproductive system is the only body system whose functions are biologically dispensable. In other words, they may be stopped without endangering a person's life. Indeed, the body will turn off the reproductive system if it perceives that other functions are immediately more important for survival. In times of stress, for example, the body will divert its energy towards overcoming the causes of the stress at the expense of the reproductive function. Hence, our sex drive may take a dive in stressful circumstances. Menstrual periods can often become irregular. With this in mind, we begin to see how the ability to reproduce becomes a privilege in the body, not a right. It also becomes evident that fertility and a balanced hormonal system is an accurate indicator of a woman's overall health.

There is a convenient way of monitoring a woman's reproductive health—by observing her menses, also known as the menstrual cycle.

The Menstrual Cycle

The menstrual cycle is like a fine symphony, a fascinating interplay of hormones and physiological responses played out by the orchestra of our magnificent body. Mother Nature prepares a woman for a potential pregnancy every cycle. A tour of the normal 28-day cycle known as the menstrual cycle will give us an appreciation of this "instrumentation."

Menstruation (Day 1)

Day 1 of your cycle is defined as the first full day of menstrual bleeding. The uterine lining built up from the preceding cycle is sloughed off and cleared away as menstrual blood. Hormone levels from the previous cycle take a sharp decline. The result is a myriad of physical and emotional symptoms commonly associated with menstruation.

Pre-Ovulation (Day 2 to 14)

The menstrual bleeding usually lasts a few days. From Day 2 on, the body is already starting to prepare itself for the next cycle. Under the influence of follicle stimulating hormone (FSH) and luteinizing hormone (LH) secreted by the pituitary gland, the follicles (fluid-filled sacs containing an egg each) in the ovaries start to manufacture and secrete estrogen. Estrogen causes the uterine lining (the endometrium) to thicken. At the same time, about 15 to 20 eggs start to mature in each ovary during this period. Each egg is encased and protected in its own follicle. The follicles also produce estrogen and other hormones including androgens. Estrogen is the hormone necessary for ovulation to occur. If ovulation occurs, in other words, if an egg is released, the level of estrogen slowly rises during this period as the uterus lining thickens and starts its preparation to receive the egg. A race begins among the follicles to become the largest. Eventually, ovulation occurs when an ovary releases an egg when the most dominant follicle bursts open.

Ovulation (Day 14 to 15)

Although it averages about two weeks, this race among the competing follicles to release an egg can take anywhere from about eight days to a month or longer to complete. The key determinant is how soon your body reaches its estrogen threshold. A high level of estrogen is required to trigger an abrupt surge of luteinizing hormone that causes the egg to literally burst through the ovary wall. This release is called ovulation.

After ovulation, the egg tumbles out into the pelvic cavity, where it is quickly transported into the fallopian tubes. The remainder of the ruptured follicle (called the corpus luteum) recedes into the ovary and begins the important task of secreting progesterone. This hormone causes blood vessels in the uterine lining to proliferate. This is done in preparation for providing nourishment for the fetus in case fertilization occurs. The increased supply of progesterone also inhibits other eggs from developing and causes the basal body temperature to rise about half a degree. Incidentally, this is the basis for determining the fertile period in your cycle with a thermometer.

Luteal Phase (Day 15 to 30)

The luteal phase is the next stage usually lasting 11 to 14 days following ovulation. In layman terms, it is the last two weeks of the menstrual cycle. It begins as the fertile period of the woman's monthly cycle.

The egg can be fertilized within 24 hours of its release, while it is still in the fallopian tubes. If the egg is fertilized, the pituitary gland produces another hormone called hCG (human chorionic gonadotropin) which causes an increased production of progesterone. This is sustained throughout the pregnancy among other changes in the expectant mother's body chemistry. The increased progesterone level in turn causes the basal body temperature to remain high throughout the luteal phase and after the 14th day. High progesterone levels are also responsible for morning sickness and other symptoms of pregnancy.

If no fertilization takes place, the progesterone level will reach its peak on day 19-22, after which the level starts to fall. If the egg is not fertilized within 24 hours, the corpus luteum starts to shrink and slow its progesterone production. Without progesterone's support, the richly-supplied uterine lining will thin out and slough off as menstruation at the end of the cycle. The uterus clears itself and prepares once again for the next cycle.

Menstrual Cycle and Hormones

Graphical representation of the menstrual cycle:

(Figure 1) shows the control by the master glands of the hypothalamus and pituitary sending follicle stimulating hormone (FSH) and luteinizing hormone (LH) to the pituitary gland.

(Figure 2) is the graph of FSH and LH levels in the blood during the cycle.

(Figure 3) shows the ebb and flow of estrogen and progesterone levels in the body.

(Figure 4) shows the thickness of the endometrial tissues over the phases of the menstrual cycle.

(Figure 5) illustrates the changes in the ovary at the various stages of the cycle when no fertilization takes place.

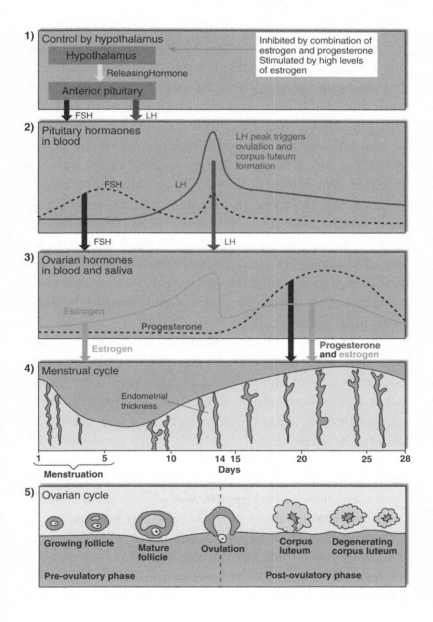

Regular Menses (Puberty to Age 45)

This menstrual cycle is a monthly affair from the onset of menses at age 12 or thereabouts. The first period marks the significant transition from child to woman and is called menarche. The exact number of days that the menstrual cycle lasts, varies from woman to woman—anywhere from 28 to 35 days. It is normally only interrupted by pregnancy.

But consider this: A hundred years ago, the average woman started her menses at age 16. She got pregnant earlier and more frequently. Without the benefit of baby formula, she lactated for longer periods to breast feed her baby. In total, women then experienced the menstrual cycle about 100 to 200 times in their lifetime. In contrast today, the average modern woman has her menarche at age 12, seldom lactates because she does not nurse her babies, have fewer children and menstruate about 350 to 400 times through their lifetime—about double our grandmothers' frequency.

It is now recognized that continual menstruation is associated with an increased occurrence of a myriad of pathological conditions including infertility, cancer, fibroids, anemia, migraines, mood shifts, abdominal pain, fluid retention and endometriosis. Against the millennia of the civilizing process, what a difference the last century made!

> It is apparent that the modern woman faces many more female-related illnesses than her counterpart just a century ago. Just what exactly is the bearing of the civilizing changes on our health? The clue lies in the hormones responsible for regulating the female menstrual cycle.

Perimenopause

Perimenopause is a transitional stage lasting between two to ten years signaling the onset of menopause. On the average, it lasts six years and begins in women between the ages of 35 and 50 years. It is a time when the woman's menses become unpredictable. The end of this stage is when the woman ceases to menstruate naturally again.

Perimenopause is brought on by the declining function of the ovaries while the woman is still going through her monthly cycles. She can find herself experiencing puzzling changes and not know why. What is actually going on in her system is a steep decrease of progesterone secretion with a more gradual decrease for estrogen. The manifestations of perimenopause can vary greatly. No two women will experience perimenopause exactly the same way. Some of the common symptoms include:

- Shorter, longer, or unpredictable menstrual cycles that get more variable the closer the woman approaches menopause
- Headaches and engorged breasts before periods
- Cramping with periods and midcycle pain
- Bleeding problems such as spotting or heavy periods
- Weight gain around the waist
- Loss of muscle tone
- Hot flushes (that will recur at menopause)
- Inexplicable depression, anxiety and apathy
- Nasal congestion and recurrent respiratory infection
- Memory loss and difficulty in thinking
- Loss of balance and dizziness
- Irritability
- Reduced sex drive

Unfortunately, perimenopause is a period when attention to hormonal balance is frequently overlooked. Women are told that there is little they can do to avert many of the symptoms that usually come on with menopause. However, this is a critical window for the women to correct their hormonal imbalance.

Menopause

The onset of menopause signals the ending of a woman's reproductive cycle. This event marks the culmination of many years of pre- and perimenopausal changes during which hormones secreted by the ovaries, namely estrogen and progesterone, decline. Menopause begins after the woman's last period and usually occurs around age 50.

The age at which menopause is triggered is linked to a number of factors. Smokers, women who are poorly nourished, and those who do not have children tend to have an earlier menopause. Menopause can be early by a few years or more due to the reduced estrogen output from the ovaries, as in the case of total hysterectomy where the uterus and ovaries are removed.

Conversely, women who are obese tend to have a later menopause because of the excess estrogen produced partly by fat cells in their system. Menopausal symptoms vary considerably from person to person too. Asians are known to have few or no symptoms other than irregular menses. Western women, however, have much higher incidences of body changes such as hot flushes, night sweats, fatigue, insomnia, breakthrough bleeding (spotting between periods), breast tenderness, vaginal dryness, painful intercourse, reduced libido, forgetfulness, joint pains, thinning of hair, heart palpitations, loss of bladder control, frequent urination, food allergies and indigestion to name just the more common ones. The resultant changes in metabolism may lead to osteoporosis, a rise in blood pressure, more fat in the blood, atherosclerosis, and an increased risk of stroke. They can give rise to depression, anxiety and irritability. The average woman gains eight pounds in the first two years of menopause. For some, these symptoms are like a living hell. Symptoms of perimenopause are often similar to those of menopause. However, they are generally more pronounced during menopause because the hormonal imbalance is more severe.

It is obviously difficult to tell exactly when menopause has set in, given the uncertain signs along the way. However a doctor can conclude that a woman has reached her menopause when she shows the following:

- FSH level in the blood higher than 50 mIU/ml (milli-international units per ml);

- Estradiol (a type of estrogen. See the section on Estrogen below) serum level less than 50 pg/ml (picograms per ml); or

- No menstruation for one full year.

A pelvic ultrasound will typically show a thin endometrium and shrunken, atrophied ovaries.

Menopause usually progresses through stages that last about ten years. The first few years signal the onset of menopause. These years are the most traumatic for the woman.

For the past 40 years, the conventional wisdom has been that menopause is caused by the absolute deficiency in estrogen. In the mistaken effort to rectify this, estrogen replacement has been prescribed to millions of women since the mid-1960s. The absolute lack of estrogen has now been shown to be an incomplete answer. As evidence of this, many women, who could not be prescribed estrogen for various reasons, found relief when treated with natural progesterone alone. Clearly, there is more to the menopausal upheaval than the simple decline in estrogen. Let us now look more closely into the female hormones to understand the issue.

Female Hormones

The two primary female hormones secreted by the ovaries are estrogen and progesterone. While each has its own functions, the biochemical actions of one offset those of the other and together they are maintained at optimal balance in a body at all times. Too much of one hormone or the other can lead to significant medical problems over time.

Estrogen

As the principal female sex hormone, estrogen affects all female sex organs, including the ovaries, cervix, fallopian tubes, vagina and breasts. It regulates the menstrual cycle, promotes cell division and is largely responsible for the development of secondary female characteristics during puberty, like the growth and development of the breasts and pubic hair. Playing its role in promoting cell growth, estrogen signals the development of the blood-rich tissues of the uterus, namely, the endometrium. This is confined to the first part of the menstrual cycle as it stimulates the maturation of the egg-containing follicle in the ovary. It softens the cervix and produces the right quality of vaginal secretion to smoothen the way for intercourse and allow the sperm to swim towards the egg. Furthermore, it is a feel-good hormone that gives women a sense of well-being.

In non-pregnant, premenopausal women, only 100-200 micrograms (µg) of estrogen are secreted daily. But during pregnancy, much more is produced.

Up till this point, we have spoken of estrogen as a single hormone. However, it is actually a complex of distinct hormones working together. The three main components are: estrone (E1), estradiol (E2) and estriol (E3). In addition, there are at least 24 other identified estrogens produced in the woman's body, and possibly more to be discovered.

We will concentrate on the main trio of estrogens for now. In healthy young women, the typical mix ratio approximates 15:15:70 respectively. This is the combination worked out by Mother Nature to be the optimum for human females.

It is important to note that there are also animal estrogens, synthetic estrogens, phytoestrogens (phyto- meaning plant) and xenoestrogens (environmental estrogens, usually from toxins such as pesticides). They belong to the same chemical family as a woman's estrogen. However, their chemical actions are less than desirable.

We have said that estrogen is a hormone that is pro-growth. Since too much of anything is generally undesirable in nature, the body has another hormone to offset and counterbalance the effects of estrogen. It is called progesterone.

Progesterone

As its name implies, progesterone is a hormone that is pro gestation. In other words, it favors the growth and well-being of the fetus. It is, thus, that without the proper amount of prog-esterone, there can be no successful pregnancy. Here is how it favors pregnancy.

One of the roles played by progesterone is to prevent further ovulation from taking place in the second half of the menstrual cycle, as earlier stated. This is when an egg has just been released, ready for fertilization to take place.

Furthermore, it causes the vaginal lining to secrete a thick mucus that is hostile to sperm and thwarts its passage into the womb once fertilization has taken place. This prevents multiple fertilizations from taking place.

To bring us back to the need to keep estrogen in check, we note that progesterone works in opposition to it. Progesterone, in fact, protects us against any uncontrolled growth-promoting effects of estrogen. It goes without saying that these two hormones must be in a good balance for the body to do well.

Progesterone is made from another hormone called pregnenolone, which in turn comes from cholesterol. Contrary to the misconception that cholesterol is absolutely bad for us, having enough good fat and cholesterol is, therefore, important for a well-functioning hormonal system. Production of progesterone occurs in several glands. In the women, it is primarily made in the ovaries just before ovulation and increases rapidly after ovulation. It is also made in the adrenal glands in both sexes and in the testes in males. In women its level is highest during the luteal phase (especially from day 19-22 of the menstrual cycle).

If fertilization does not take place after ovulation, the secretion of progesterone decreases and menstruation occurs 12 to 14 days later under normal conditions. If fertilization does occur, progesterone is greatly increased during pregnancy through its secretion by the placenta. The increased level of progesterone acts to prevent spontaneous abortion and keep the pregnancy intact.

About 20-25 mg of progesterone is produced per day during a woman's monthly cycle. Up to 300-400 mg are produced daily during pregnancy. This is evidence of the importance of progesterone during pregnancy.

Estrogen Effect vs. Progesterone Effect

As mentioned earlier, progesterone acts as a moderator to estrogen. For example, estrogen enhances salt and water retention while progesterone is a natural diuretic, removing water from the system by inducing urination. Estrogen stimulates breast cysts while progesterone protects against breast cysts. Furthermore, estrogen has been associated with breast and endometrial cancers, while progesterone has a cancer-preventive effect.

> Studies have shown that premenopausal women who were deficient in progesterone had 5.4 times the risk of breast cancer compared to healthy women.

Having stated this, it is important to note that both these hormones are necessary for the body to function optimally. Progesterone will not work without some estrogen in the body to prime the pump, as it were. The following table illustrates how progesterone and estrogen balance each other.

Estrogen Effect	Progesterone Effect
Causes endometrium to proliferate	Maintains secretory endometrium
Stimulates formation of breast tissues; may lead to fibrocystic breast or breast cancer	Protects against fibrocystic breast and prevents breast cancer
	Helps convert fat to energy
Increases body fat	Prevents endometrial cancer
Increases endometrial-cancer risk	
Increase gallbladder disease risk	Promotes bone growth
	Restores vascular tone
Slight effect in preventing bone loss	Normalize blood clot risk
Increases blood clot risk	

Figure 1. Estrogen and Progesterone Effects: a Comparison

Summary

Estrogen and progesterone are the two key regulatory hormones for the female menstrual and reproductive cycle. Their levels change constantly during the menstrual cycle and also during the life cycle as a woman matures and finally reaches menopause. They oppose each other, maintaining a body that is balanced hormonally to provide optimal function. Estrogen is pro-growth and excessive levels of it can trigger a host of diseases.

Progesterone offsets estrogen and this, as we will see, is a key hormone often deficient in women of the modern world. When hormones are well balanced, women have a sense of well-being and pass easily through the monthly menstrual cycle into menopause without health problems. This is the way Nature designed it. Only when the hormonal balance is upset do symptoms and disease arise.

Chapter 3

Hormonal Imbalance

What Upsets The Estrogen Balance?

We concluded in the previous chapter that our body needs both estrogen and progesterone in the right quantities to function healthily. Generally, when our regulatory systems are well maintained, a state of perfect harmony will result among the components of the systems—a state known as homeostasis.

It is time for us to investigate the ills that befall anyone who loses the fine balance between the mutually-moderating hormones, in particular, estrogen and progesterone. You will see that estrogen, when present in excess in our system, leads to a condition identified as estrogen dominance.

At the very beginning, we asserted that much of the ill-health suffered today is the result of an increasingly unhealthy environment. Before the industrial revolution, the changes that humans made to this earth were never drastic in their scope, severity, or suddenness. Almost always, Nature was allowed time to repair these assaults.

With the advent of our industrial society 100 years ago, the self-healing capacity of the earth has gradually been destroyed. At the same time, the science of chemistry was discovered and applied to industry with all enthusiasm. It brought untold wealth to new industrialists. Never before in our history had so many new and toxic chemicals been created supposedly for our benefit. In truth, many of these creations undermined the world's health. Not only are some of these toxic beyond imagination, they are also so persistent that they continue to post a threat to our health long after they have been released into the environment. It took many tragic deaths and much suffering to awaken us to the hazards of our exotic chemicals. Yes, society has advanced by great leaps, but it has come at a great price as well.

The unfortunate effects of environmental pollution on our hormones alone are a frightening example of their far-reaching consequences. We will consider some of these and see how they get into our system to set the health time-bomb ticking.

The most obvious route is through our diet. Tradition has it that we are what we eat. Thanks to the demands of our faster pace of life we have taken to eating foods that are reconstituted, stabilized and loaded with preservatives. Chemical agents are added which our forebears never had to put in their mouths. In just one century, we have managed to turn our diet from fresh fruits and whole foods to fast and processed heat-and-eat meals.

Moreover, agriculture has moved from traditional time-tested methods to practices that put a premium on the speed of production. The backbone of their approach is to bring the livestock to the market as soon as possible. Chemicals have been introduced into the industry for this purpose. These chemicals eventually find their way into the human body. Some of these have estrogen-like properties that kick off the long-term ills associated with a chronic excess of estrogen. Such estrogen-like compounds in the environment are termed xenoestrogens (Xeno is the Greek word for foreign or strange), sometimes as xenobiotics or xenohormones. These terms have been used interchangeably. Chemicals displaying this ability to mimic estrogen are described as xenoestrogenic.

The truth is that the modern environment is hazardous to our health. Women in non-industrialized cultures whose diets are still based on whole foods remain untainted even today. They seldom suffer a deficiency in proges-terone or the ravages of excess estrogen manifested as menopausal symptoms.

While hormonal imbalance was a rare disorder 50 years ago, today it is nearly an epidemic. It is now rare for women not to suffer from hormonal imbalance at some point or other in their life. If you live in the developed world, in or near a metropolitan city, you are almost sure to suffer some form of hormonal imbalance, especially estrogen dominance.

Estrogen, the Deadly Intruder

1. Drugs in commercially raised livestock

Traditionally, cattle were raised on grass, hay and natural organic fodder. Chickens were allowed to run free and forage or fed with corn from the fields. They only ate what nature meant for them to eat. This is in stark contrast to the feed of commer-cialized cattle and poultry of today. The animals are put on a fast track of growth for economic reasons. So they are routinely given feed laced with, among other things, pesticides and hormones, both of which have estrogen-like properties. These pesticides "protect" the feed and the hormones accelerate the animals' development. This strategy has a very dramatic impact on the farm's output. It only takes six weeks to grow a chicken to market size now– compared to 16 weeks in 1940.

In addition, the economic losses that accompany any disease outbreak in farms are unthinkable. Also for economy of space and convenience of husbandry, the livestock are often cooped very close together. Up to 80,000 birds may be packed into one warehouse. As this is a recipe for an epidemic, a disaster to the farmers, they take the precaution of dosing the animals with antibiotics and other drugs to keep disease at bay. It is interesting to note that one half of all antibiotics in the United States are used in raising livestock—25 million pounds a year! The use of antibiotics is especially prevalent in poultry farms. However, these antibiotics and drugs can disrupt the hormones in our body. One of the unintended effects is an excess of estrogen in the consumer's body.

As a precaution, we recommend that you trim off the fat and skin from poultry and fish as these fatty tissues tend to store the hormones and drugs. Incidentally fish is a far safer meat than beef or chicken in terms of hormone load.

Deep-sea fish such as halibut, sardines, cod and mackerel are better, being more isolated from the pollutants in coastal waters.

2. Pesticides in fruits and vegetables

When was the last time you saw a wormy or blighted apple in the supermarket? You probably cannot recall as it was a very long ago. The reason isn't hard to guess. Your supermarket only sells the most appealing produce. Perfect appearance has replaced good nutrition as the criterion for buying food. To keep the fruits and vegetables unblemished, farmers douse them with pesticides. So if you buy them in any developed country, you end up eating a lot of pesticides.

The troublesome synthetic pesticides include insecticides, herbicides, fungicides and nematocides. About 70 percent of the pesticides used are applied to crops and livestock. One group of insecticides is called organochlorines, with DDT (dichloro-diphenyltrichloroethane) being the most well-known.

We sometimes ingest the chemicals even when these plant-protecting agents are not sprayed on the fruits or vegetables themselves. They might come from a distant source and contaminate the soil or water, ending up in the honest farmers' land. They are so stable chemically that they can persist long enough to be absorbed by the plants and make their way into the produce that we eat.

Despite efforts to stop this practice, pesticides are still illegally applied. So it is a small consolation that the USA has banned dangerous pesticides such as DDT. It is still being freely applied in poor producer countries. South American and African growers are often implicated. Economic imperatives drive them to knowingly use illegal pesticides. Thanks to the globalized world the fruits of their labor find their way to our table. The USDA recommends that we eat five servings of fruits and vegetables a day. It is estimated that this recommendation exposes a person to such illegal pesticides about 75 times a year if the produce are purchased in regular supermarkets.

Just how big is the danger? Approximately five billion pounds of pesticides, herbicides, fungicides and other biocides are being added to the world each year. It is estimated that in the past hundred years, several hundred billion pounds of pesticides have been released into the environment. Remembering that hormones are secreted and act in very minute quantities, you will appreciate the fact that we have enough contaminants to ruin our health many times over.

According to *A Shopper's Guide to Pesticides in Produce*, strawberries (contain vinclozolin, a known endocrine disruptor), bell peppers, peaches, apples, apricots and spinach are the most contaminated. Foods with the least amount of pesticides include avocados, corn, onions, sweet potatoes, banana, green onions, broccoli and cauliflower. If you are eating non-organic fruits and vegetables, we suggest that you wash them well with diluted vinegar and peel them. This will help to eliminate pesticides on the skin. Needless to say, this will not get rid of the pesticides inside. Similarly, discard the outer leaves of leafy vegetables.

3. Xenoestrogens in petrochemicals

A good percentage of the petroleum pumped from the ground is converted to industrially useful chemicals instead of gasoline. The resultant petrochemical compounds are found in consumer products such as creams, lotions, soaps, shampoos, perfumes, hair sprays and deodorizers. Such compounds are often xenoestrogens as well. Unknowingly, we cover ourselves with solutions that contribute to the hormonal imbalance within. And the most obvious source of petroleum-derived xenoestrogens must be exhaust fumes from cars and other combustion engines.

In recent years, there has been a drive towards producing and using biodegradable items. This initiative strives to solve the world's pollution problems. The problems are amplified by chemicals that defy Nature's attempts at breaking them down into their harmless components again. One of the most toxic and difficult classes of xenoestrogenic pollutants known is the persistent organic pollutants or POPs. They are highly resistant to chemical degradation and, therefore, last a long time. Polychlorinated biphenyls (PCB), DDT and a wide variety of man-made chemicals fall into this class. They have a strong affinity for fat and, as a result, accumulate in increasing concentration with each step up the food chain.

A number of chemicals used to make plastics are known to be xenoestrogenic as well. One example is the phthalates, a class of over 50 related chemicals used to make plastics more flexible and durable. One of them, diethylhexyl phthalate, is an additive used in PVC (polyvinyl chloride) that goes into making rainwear, footwear, upholstery materials, shower curtains, floor tiles, blood bags, heat-seal coating on metal foils (such as those found on yogurt containers) and in certain types of inks and pesticides.

Another, diethyl phthalate, is commonly used in blister packing and in numerous items such as nail polish, insect repellents, adhesives, toys, car components and toothbrushes.

Inevitably, some of the phthalate finds its way into our body through foods that have absorbed these chemicals from their packaging or from their manufacturing process. There is evidence that this happens to chocolate bars, potato chips, soft cheeses, cakes packaged in paper and cardboard, vegetable burger mix, vegetable fat and sausages.

4. Organic solvents

A common source of industrial xenoestrogens often overlooked is a family of chemicals called solvents. As the name suggests, they are liquids in which some principal ingredient is dissolved. They are overlooked because they are usually not identified on the packaging. It is the main ingredient that is advertised—spray paints, nail varnish, perfumes and such. Thus we allow these solvents to enter our body through the skin and quickly accumulate in the fat (adipose) layer or fat-rich tissues such as our nerve sheaths (myelin).

The common organic solvents include alcohols, aldehydes, glycols and ketones. They are commonly found in cosmetics, nail varnish and nail varnish remover, glues, paints, varnishes and other types of finishes, cleaning products like those for dry-cleaning and carpets and infused in fiberboard and other processed timber.

5. Hormone Replacement Therapy (HRT)

Since the mid-1940s, millions of women have been prescribed estrogen as the way to prevent menopausal symptoms. Such estrogens are synthetic and made in the laboratory. They are predominantly estradiol, a form of estrogen that, in excess, is not welcomed by the body. Fortunately, the deadly side effects of HRT have now been exposed. Study after study now conclude that such HRT using synthetic estrogen such as Pempro®, Pemarin® and a host of other such related drugs increases the risk of cancer, heart disease, not to mention minor side effects such as bloatedness, headaches, and depression, just to name a few.

6. Ovarian cysts or tumors

Excess estrogen can arise from ovarian cysts or tumors. This is a silent but common cause of disorders in the body. That goes unnoticed until the disorder becomes troublesome. If the patient suffers the symptoms stoically, the discovery often comes too late for effective treatment.

7. Stress

While everybody knows that emotional stress affects our mood and energy levels, the actual mechanism is less apparent. A little stress with a little adrenaline rush now and then is relatively harmless. In fact, it has been said to be good for us. But prolonged stress is another matter altogether. The trouble begins when chronic stress causes adrenal gland fatigue. Stress triggers the release of cortisol, the body's antistress hormone. However, cortisol suppresses the production of progesterone.

Over a period of prolonged stress, the reduced level of progesterone tilts the estrogen-progesterone balance in favor of estrogen. This estrogen dominance in turn causes insomnia and anxiety, which further taxes the adrenal gland to put out more cortisol. It sets off another round in the vicious cycle. After a few years, the adrenal gland becomes exhausted and cannot work up any more cortisol. This dysfunction leads to blood sugar imbalance, other hormonal imbalances and chronic fatigue.

8. Obesity

The good news is that fat has a definite role in our diet. Estrogen and progesterone are both hormones that are produced in the body naturally. It is now known that the process requires cholesterol as a building block. Without cholesterol, estrogen and progesterone levels will be reduced. The higher the fat intake, the higher the conversion of fat to estrogen will be. However, there is a limit to the good that this does for us. While fat is necessary for hormone production, excessive fat consumption increases the risk of estrogen dominance.

The world today is aware that overeating is the norm in developed countries. Over 50 Percent of all adults in America are overweight. The population in first-world countries, especially in the Western hemisphere, derives a large part of its dietary calorie from sugar. At the same time, their women have a much higher incidence of menopausal symptoms associated with an excess of estrogen.

Conversely, studies have shown that estrogen and progesterone levels fell in women who switched from a typical high saturated-fat, refined-carbohydrate diet to a low-fat, high-fiber and plant-based diet even though they did not adjust their total calorie intake. It has been put down to the fact that plants contain over 5,000 known sterols that have progestrogenic effects. People who eat more whole foods have a far lower incidence of menopausal symptoms because their pre- and post-menopause levels of estrogen do not drop as significantly.

9. Liver dysfunction

A habit which is enjoyed at the expense of health in many rich countries is drinking alcoholic beverages. As with so many other pleasures, over-indulgence is the real villain. A persistently high concentration of alcohol in the bloodstream puts an intolerable stress on the liver, which is the main organ for disposing of toxins and unwanted proteins including hormones.

Liver diseases such as cirrhosis, arising from the abuse of alcohol, reduce the rate at which the liver breaks down estrogen. Taking drugs that can impair liver function may also contribute to a higher level of estrogen. The prescribing doctor owes it to the patient to ascertain that estrogen dominance will not add to the patient's problems.

10. Deficiency in Vitamin B6 and Magnesium

In the natural course of our body's chemistry, hormones are replaced in cycles. As part of this cycle, used estrogen is eliminated as a new supply is secreted. The neutralization of estrogen occurs in the liver and the process requires two other important ingredients: vitamin B6 and magnesium. It is one of the potential vicious cycles to watch out for.

Too little of these two nutrients will result in too much estrogen floating about in the system. Too much estrogen will worsen the deficiency in magnesium and the B vitamins.

It is a situation that is easily rectified with the right supplementation. Magnesium is a natural muscle relaxant and calming agent. It comes as no surprise then that those suffering from too much estrogen often have accompanying insomnia, chronic fatigue and fibromyalgia.

11. Increase in caffeine consumption

Coffee drinking is another controversial social habit. It is difficult to believe that the aromatic brew loved all over the world has a dark secret—caffeine. Caffeine intake from all sources had been linked with higher estrogen levels regardless of the person's age, body mass index (BMI), or other attributes. Studies have shown that women who consume at least 500 mg (milligrams) of caffeine daily, the equivalent of four or five cups of coffee, have nearly 70 percent more estrogen during the early follicular phase than women who consume no more than 100 mg of caffeine, or less than one cup of coffee daily. Although it is not the only drink to pack this stimulant, coffee is the most common beverage to contain as much of it, ounce for ounce. Tea is not much better as it contains about half the amount of caffeine in coffee. The wiser choice would be herbal teas like chamomile that contain no caffeine.

Summary

Living in the modern world today carries many hazards in terms of estrogen overload. We are literally bathed in a sea of estrogen. From caffeine to stress, to plastic containers and shampoos that we are so used to as part of everyday life.

There is no easy escape from all the causal factors. Yet these are the very factors contributing to estrogen overload. While any single factor may not be significant, the total sum of the exposure to many if not all of the above will, over time, trigger off a chronic condition associated with a body flooded with estrogen.

Chapter 4

Types of Hormonal Imbalance

While we virtually live in a sea of environmental estrogen, not all of us have symptoms of hormonal imbalance. The reason is that no two persons are exactly alike. Other factors of personal makeup account for the extent of the symptoms suffered. Those who are thin and have good liver function are better equipped to process and convert any excess estrogen into inactive byproducts (called metabolites), thereby reducing their estrogen load.

Obesity, on the other hand, increases estrogen production from the fat cells and provides the fat tissues that store the excess hormone. It is worth repeating that a chronically high level of blood alcohol can impair liver function in the body. All of these factors aggravate the estrogen dominance.

Female hormonal balance requires the delicate modulation of estrogen, progesterone and androgens. Imbalances among these hormones can be categorized in three different ways: progesterone deficiency, estrogen deficiency and estrogen excess.

1. Progesterone Deficiency

There is no doubt that you would have heard complaints among friends that sound very much like:

- My period just does not come.
- My periods come irregularly.
- I get scared when I see large clots during my period.
- My breasts hurt when I am hugged.

- I cannot fit into my shoes because of water retention.
- I have a cyst in my breast.
- I have fibroids.
- I have endometriosis.

For reasons that we have explained, these complaints are more persistent in urban areas and busy cities. They are all signs of progesterone deficiency. Along with the specific complaints listed, there are frequently also the symptoms of PMS, insomnia, early miscarriage, infertility, unexplained weight gain and anxiety.

This is, in fact, the most common category of hormonal imbalance among women of all ages. Progesterone is absolutely necessary to keep the effects of estrogen in check. Without sufficient progesterone, estrogen wreaks havoc on the woman. She may suffer infrequent periods (oligomenorrhea), or have none at all (amenorrhea). If periods do occur, they can be overly heavy. This is due to tissue buildup in the uterus from prolonged progesterone deficiency. A few days before the period comes, women deficient in progesterone often report PMS symptoms. PMS can last from a few days to as long as two weeks, from the time of ovulation (day 14) to the onset of the next period (day 28). The more severe the deficiency, the longer the PMS lasts.

It is clear, from the list of complaints above that progesterone deficiency symptoms also include cystic breasts, painful breasts, endometriosis and fibroids. In addition, most women deficient in progesterone feel irritated and anxious. They often visit their doctor complaining about difficulty of sleeping and relaxing, or feeling like a nervous wreck.

The symptoms of progesterone deficiency are similar to those of estrogen dominance, as we shall see below. The culprit is an estrogen overload when progesterone is not present in sufficient quantities. Correction should focus on reducing estrogen and supplementing with natural progesterone, as we shall discuss in greater detail later. The common-sense first step is to cut off any further intake of estrogen, for example, discontinue taking birth control pills. Applying a natural progesterone cream can increase the progesterone level. We will talk more about remedies later.

2. Estrogen Deficiency

It is equally common to hear middle-age women complain of the following recurring set of worries:

- I'm afraid I'm losing my mind.
- I cannot remember my grandchildren's birthdays.
- I'm so depressed I feel the world is crumbling around me.
- I don't know how I am going to face tomorrow.
- I feel a heat wave spreading through my body.
- I wake up soaking in sweat.
- I am not lubricating well during intercourse.
- I have lost my appetite for sex.
- I feel tired all day long.
- I can't fall asleep.
- My breasts are suddenly sagging.
- I am gaining weight very quickly.
- I feel bloated like a balloon.

Symptoms like night sweats, hot flushes, sagging breasts, vaginal dryness, painful intercourse, osteoporosis, fibrocystic lumps, mood swings, depression and memory loss flag the problem of a diminishing output of estrogen, a feel-good hormone for women.

If you are observant, you will pick out a pattern of ups and downs that should warn you of a deficiency in estrogen. They are:

- **A sense of well-being from day 7 to 14.** Estrogen hits its highest level from day 12 to day 21. If you don't feel good during this period, your body is telling you that you need more estrogen.

- **During the few days before and during your period, the symptoms are at their most severe.** The discomforts feel the worst as this corresponds to the phase in your monthly cycle when the estrogen level in your body is at its lowest.

- **You feel better during pregnancy after the first trimester, when most women feel worse.** Women with a normal estrogen-progesterone balance before pregnancy usually feel the ill-effects of estrogen level surges in this stage. Conversely, the one who is normally short of estrogen will enjoy the boost in estrogen level during the first trimester of the pregnancy.

- **When you are on contraceptive pills, you feel better.** The pill is just a dose of estrogen. If popping them improves your condition then it indicates that your estrogen level was low prior to starting on the pill.

This hormone imbalance is most common in menopausal women, especially with petite or slim women. As you will see below, there is a reverse effect for overweight women.

The approach to correcting this set of symptoms is to enhance the estrogen level in the system. Estrogen replacement using drugs such as Premarin® is an accepted means of alleviating the symptoms. But it must be accompanied by natural progesterone if side effects are to be avoided. A far better way is to increase estrogen level with natural compounded estrogen such as *Bi-est®* or *Tri-est®* in conjunction with natural progesterone cream. The full remedial regime will be discussed in Part 2 of this book.

3. Estrogen Excess:

It is hardly surprising to see that the symptoms caused by a deficiency in progesterone should resemble those arising from an excess of estrogen. After all, it is progesterone that moderates the estrogen. Typical complaints that we hear from women whose systems are awash with estrogen include:

- My breasts are painful and tender to touch.
- My breasts are swollen and getting bigger.
- I can't put on my rings.
- My legs are swollen around the ankles.
- I am getting cramps again like when I was teenager.
- My period flows are heavier than normal.
- I am getting more impatient.
- People tell me I am too bossy.

Symptoms of bloating, rapid weight gain, heavy bleeding, migraine headaches, foggy thinking, insomnia, hot flushes and breast tenderness during the first two weeks of the menstrual cycle are common among sufferers. The excess estrogen will thicken the endometrium more than normal. Then, this thick uterine lining will be shed as copious, sometimes clotted, blood when the period arrives. The greater-than-normal effort required to expel the thick mass results in pain or cramping in the lower pelvic area.

Let us look for the patterns that can be explained in terms of an estrogen oversupply:

- **You feel better from day 14 to 28 of the cycle.**
  This is the time of peak progesterone secretion with progesterone counteracting the excess estrogen that helps you naturally feel better.

- **You feel worse during pregnancy than before.** During pregnancy, your estrogen level increases. If you feel worse, chances are you already have a relatively high estrogen level before the pregnancy and the body has little tolerance for the increase occasioned by the pregnancy.

Only about five percent of women produce a naturally high level of estrogen. So they are a very small minority in this category. More often than not, the excess estrogen is the result of a HRT program or contraceptive pills. It may sometimes be the presence of benign ovarian cysts.

Unlike estrogen deficiency, the effect of which is more immediate, symptoms of estrogen over-abundance develop more slowly, often over three to five years. Interestingly, the mental functions of these women are not affected and they remain very sharp with good memory. Obese women are the most prone to this condition as opposed to estrogen-deficient women who tend to be small-framed or underweight.

The problem is overcome if the patient discontinues HRT that uses synthetic estrogen alone (which is termed estrogen replacement therapy or ERT). Similarly, other means of contraception than using estrogen should be employed. Recovering normal body weight is a priority for those who are obese. A more thorough discussion of the remedies will follow in Part 2 below.

4. Androgen (Male Hormone) Excess:

It might surprise some women to learn that the female endocrine system does secrete a small amount of male hormones called androgens. An example is testosterone, which is required for the optimum function of a woman's body by maintaining her energy level and sex drive. However, when the androgen levels exceed the normal range, complications do arise. Common complaints among women who have the condition are:

- I am breaking out in pimples like an adolescent.
- My hair is falling out by the handful.
- I feel very aggressive.
- I have a noticeable mustache.

The more extreme symptoms will include acne, polycystic ovary syndrome (PCOS), excess facial and body hair, thinning hair on the head, infertility and midcycle pain.

The excessive intake of sugar and simple carbohydrates in the diet often brings on the symptoms. It has been shown that excess sugar stimulates androgen receptors located outside the ovary, leading to the increased androgenic symptoms mentioned above. The androgen will lock in with the receptors and block the release of eggs from the follicle, causing polycystic ovary disease. As androgen is a male hormone, it is no surprise that such women display the male attributes of aggressiveness, baldness on the head (a specific condition termed male pattern baldness), excess facial and body hair as well as acne.

Polycystic ovary disease is often accompanied by insulin resistance and glucose intolerance, both precursors to diabetes, and those suffering from PCOS often suffer from diabetes as well. It is common, therefore, to treat PCOS with diabetic medication.

In addition, doctors recommend a dietary adjustment of reducing sugar and grains accompanied with a proper exercise regimen. Natural progesterone cream can be applied to restore hormonal balance and discontinued when symptoms are resolved. If progesterone level rises each month during the luteal phase of the cycle, the normal synchronal pattern of estrogen and progesterone is maintained and excessive androgen seldom occurs.

5. Estrogen Dominance (Relative Low Progesterone)

An earlier section briefly mentioned the complementary relation between estrogen and progesterone as a control mechanism within the woman's body. Too much estrogen or too little progesterone will result in a condition we term estrogen dominance. The condition is manifested through complaints that combine the lists of complaints found in the case of progesterone deficiency as well as an excess of estrogen above.

Other possible symptoms include:

- Acceleration of the aging process.
- Hypoglycemia (low sugar level in the blood).
- Premenopausal bone loss.
- Osteoporosis.
- Thyroid dysfunction.
- Uterine cancer and fibroids.

There are variations to the causes of estrogen dominance. These will be explained as scenarios leading up to the symptoms.

Estrogen and progesterone work in synchronization with each other as a check-and-balance to achieve hormonal harmony in all our bodies. It is not the absolute quantities of estrogen or progesterone but rather the relative abundance of estrogen over progesterone that is the main cause of health problems when they are off balance.

The output of sex hormones, including estrogen and progesterone, declines gradually with age. In contrast, there is a drastic change in the rate of decline in these two hormones during the perimenopausal and menopausal years for the women mentioned earlier.

From age 35 to 50, there is a 75 percent reduction in the production of progesterone in the body. Estrogen, during the same period, only declines about 35 percent. By menopause, the total amount of progesterone produced is extremely low, while estrogen is still present in the body at about half its premenopausal level.

With the gradual drop in estrogen but severe drop in progesterone, there is insufficient progesterone to counteract the amount of estrogen in a woman's body. Many women in their mid-thirties, most women during perimenopause (mid-forties) and essentially all women during menopause (age 50 and beyond) are overloaded with estrogen and at the same time suffering from progesterone deficiency because of the severe drop in physiological production during this period. The end result is excessive estrogen relative to progesterone, a condition we call estrogen dominance.

According to the late Dr. John Lee, the world's authority on natural hormone therapy, the key to hormonal balance is the modulation of the progesterone to estrogen ratio. For optimum health, the physiological progesterone to estrogen ratio should be between 200 and 300 to 1.

The following graph (Figure 6, not to scale) shows the fall in the production of estrogen and progesterone in a woman's body over time.

Estrogen Dominance in Premenopausal Women

There are two periods in a woman's life when her progesterone level is naturally low—once at puberty and again at perimenopause, the few years right before menopause. In the intervening years between puberty and perimenopause, known as premenopause, the production of progesterone can go awry, leading to estrogen dominance. Two common causes, anovulation and luteal malfunction, have been cited for this.

A. Anovulation

Ovulation is the time of the monthly cycle when an ovarian follicle releases an ovum or egg. Under normal circumstances, the released egg makes it way from the ovary to the uterus, ready for fertilization. This usually happens from day 12 to day 14 of the menstrual cycle. After the egg is released, the empty follicle becomes the corpus luteum. This is the "laboratory" that produces progesterone.

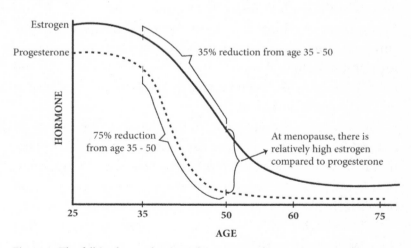

Figure 6. The fall in the production of estrogen and progesterone in a woman's body over time.

When the follicles become dysfunctional, no eggs are released, a condition called anovulation. If a woman is not ovulating, there would not be a corpus luteum to produce progesterone. Clinical measurements will show both low estrogen and low progesterone levels. Though low in absolute terms, the estrogen will still be higher in proportion. The symptoms associated with estrogen dominance, like PMS, mood swings, cramps and tender breast, eventually surface. Many women are unsuspectingly afflicted as they still have a seemingly normal menstrual cycle. Anovulation is commonly caused by the exposure of female embryos to the environmental estrogens (also called xenobiotics or xenoestrogens) discussed earlier. It is also correlated to a poor diet and stress.

B. Luteal malfunction

More common than anovulation is a condition where the egg is produced but the corpus luteum malfunctions by failing to make enough progesterone. Laboratory measurements will show a high estrogen but low progesterone level and symptoms typical of estrogen dominance would arise. Without adequate progesterone, the chances of achieving pregnancy are reduced. Don't forget that progesterone causes the blood vessels in the endometrial tissues to proliferate. This maintains the womb and nourishes the fetus that results when the egg is fertilized. Thus, infertility and spontaneous abortions are indicative of this condition called luteal malfunction.

Estrogen Dominance In Menopausal Women
According To Dr. John Lee

Dr. John Lee, author of the book *Progesterone: The multiple roles of a remarkable hormone*, has treated thousands of menopausal women in the 1980s and 1990s with a program that was contrary to popular medical thinking at the time. Instead of prescribing estrogen alone, the standard of medical practice then, Dr. Lee prescribed natural progesterone alone for treatment of many menopausal symptoms. In addition to relieving the menopausal symptoms, the treatment was able to reverse osteoporosis and prevent cancer. Studies have confirmed that this approach has vast palliative effects, helping about 60 to 80 percent of the patients afflicted with menopausal symptoms.

The key to Dr. Lee's approach lies in understanding the balance between estrogen and progesterone.

According to him, what is commonly misinterpreted as an absolute deficiency in estrogen during the menopausal years is, in effect, estrogen dominance, caused by an extremely low progesterone level. During menopause, progesterone production falls to approximately one percent of its premenopausal level. In comparison, the production of estrogen falls by about 50 percent going into menopause. The disproportionate reduction leaves very little progesterone to oppose the still significant level of postmenopausal estrogen. The toxic effect of estrogen dominance results in the myriad of distressful symptoms.

In the West, the population affected by the estrogen dominance syndrome approaches half of all women over age 35, as they enter the transitional phase of child-bearing life (until age 45). As severity of the symptoms and the patients' tolerance can vary to a large degree, a more reliable diagnosis should be carried out to determine if the patient's estrogen is in relative excess.

Definitive diagnosis can be made through a thorough examination of the patient and her medical history, accompanied by laboratory tests of estrogen and progesterone levels. However, few doctors actually do this. Worse yet, they sometimes aggravate the patient's symptoms by following "accepted" practice and prescribing more estrogen.

Dr. Lee's treatment is remarkably simple and makes logical sense—since estrogen dominance is the root of the problem, reduce the estrogen to progesterone ratio by increasing progesterone. When the opposing effect of progesterone is increased, the toxic effect of estrogen is decreased. Consequently, many women who followed this protocol were able to reduce their menopausal symptoms remarkably.

Hormone Replacement Treatment

Menopause is often thought of as a time when the balance between the hormones estrogen and progesterone in the system is upset. The symptoms, from hot flushes to vaginal dryness to water retention to mood swings, osteoporosis and memory lapses, are well known.

In 1964, estrogen replacement therapy (ERT) was first promulgated as a cure for hormonal imbalance. It was backed by the pharmaceutical industry which sold a synthetic estrogen oral supplement called Premarin®. With the drug, symptoms of menopause were greatly reduced. It was hailed as the miracle drug to help menopausal women live the life they were living before. There is now little doubt that menopause is not solely due to estrogen deficiency. However, very few doctors knew this at the time.

Eventually, many women on ERT discovered that they were accumulating fat on their hips and abdomen. They were also more prone to osteoporosis, loss of sex drive and swollen breasts.

It sent researchers back to the lab for more trials. They tried other synthetic hormones in combination. The drugs, sold under trade names of Provera® and the like, are well-used examples.

The trials yielded inconsistent results because they were missing the point. Synthetic hormones used in the so-called hormone replacement therapy (HRT) often resemble the body's hormones but do not have the same effect. Worse than that, they sometimes have undesirable side effects. *The Journal of the American Medical Association* (JAMA) published the Chen study from Washington, reporting that five years of HRT almost doubles the risk of breast cancer compared to non-users. Another issue is that JAMA found no evidence in a 6.8 year follow-up study to support the claim that Premarin® protected users from heart disease compared to non-users.

In 2002, the journal further published the stunning findings from the federally funded Women's Health Initiative (WHI) of more than 16,000 women. This study put to rest the HRT controversy and dashed the hopes of many who were taking the hormones estrogen and progestin in their synthetic form after menopause.

This well-funded study of the two-hormone combination was stopped three years early when it was found to increase the risk for breast cancer. In addition, women on the treatment suffered more heart attacks, more strokes and more life-threatening blood clots than those who were given a placebo.

On the basis of these findings, it is imperative that the use of estrogen-only prescriptions like Premarin® or combination estrogen-progestin drugs such as Pempro® should be reassessed. While the use of such drugs still has its place in selective cases, blanket prescription of the drug would be unconscionable. So how do 50 million menopausal women find relief from the symptoms? Interestingly, clinical experience has shown that women who were postmenopausal but not on ERT found relief from their distressing symptoms when they used natural progesterone alone. Clearly, there is more to the menopausal picture than just a deficiency in estrogen alone. Replacement with synthetic estrogen with or without progestin is not the answer.

Summary

Imbalances of estrogen and progesterone in our body can lead to a variety of symptoms. It is important to recognize the deficiency type, as the manifestations and treatments differ for each one. Count it our good fortune that the common denominators among most of today's woes have been identified. It is an excess of estrogen relative to an absolute deficiency in progesterone. For simplicity, this is termed estrogen dominance. This is commonly seen in those who are overweight. In the absence of external factors that cause an increase in estrogen such as a course of HRT or having a tubal ligation, obesity alone is the most important factor. Those who are thin seldom suffer estrogen dominance and frequently are estrogen-deficient. Let us now look into the myriad of symptomatic expressions of estrogen dominance.

Chapter 5

Estrogen Dominance Continuum

By now, it should be clear that estrogen dominance is the underlying common factor for a variety of common illnesses and syndromes suffered by women. Whereas they were thought to be unrelated health complaints before, we now know that they are, in fact, different manifestations of the same unresolved underlying root cause. The difference is only in the particular tissues or organs of a woman's body that are impacted by it and also the patient's constitution. As with most health factors, there is no distinct line between how much estrogen is healthy and how much is hazardous. We therefore think of it as being a continuum. Different amounts of it over different lengths of time may result in different manifestations at different periods in one's life. The estrogen dominance continuum is a state of having an excess of estrogen relative to progesterone in one's system throughout one's lifetime, with different manifestations at different stages of that lifetime.

It should not surprise us that the list of illnesses linked to estrogen dominance should overlap those associated with a deficiency or excess of one or other sex hormones discussed earlier. The long list below is not comprehensive but it gives us an idea of the troubles that estrogen dominance can trigger. Let us now look at each of these in more detail.

1. Endometriosis

Endometriosis is very common even if it is not well recognized. Statistics has it that approximately 10 to15 percent of women in their reproductive years, from age 25 to 45, are affected. About 30 percent of affected women are infertile. It is a condition where endometrial tissues are found in locations outside the uterus. The parts where this can occur are the ovaries, fallopian tubes, vagina, abdomen, deep inside the uterine muscle, the bowel, bladder, utero-sacral ligaments (ligaments that hold the uterus in place), peritoneum (the membrane lining the pelvic and abdominal cavity), or other parts of the body. It can also grow between organs and cause them to stick together. The endometrial tissue causing the disorder is essentially the same as the tissue that lines the uterus. It grows under the influence of estrogen and may be sloughed off during menstruation just like tissues in the uterus.

The causes of endometriosis are not yet fully understood. There are quite a few theories. Their theoretical bases range from genetics to our toxic environment. Backward bleeding, or retrograde menstruation, when menstrual blood flows up into the uterus instead of down, is thought to be the leading cause. Many researchers believe that estrogens and their close relatives, the xenoestrogens, play a significant causative role in this disorder. This theory would fit our assertion all along. Since endometrial cells are estrogen-responsive, any time there is estrogen dominance, they tend to proliferate.

Although our knowledge of what causes endometriosis is incomplete, your risk of developing it seems to increase with the following factors:

- Family history of endometriosis. It is especially high when a mother or sister has the condition.

- Late childbearing. In general, conceiving after age 30 is correlated with endometriosis.

- History of long menstrual cycles with a shorter than normal time between cycles.

- Abnormal uterus structure. This has to do with retrograde menstruation, perhaps.

- Diet high in hydrogenated fat (especially the variety termed trans-fat). Oily foods cooked at high temperatures, such as French fries or cookies, are implicated.

- Stress. This would explain why the condition is more common in cities than sedate rural backwaters.

The most common symptoms are pain and cramps that coincide with the menstrual cycle. Scar tissue may form wherever the endometrial tissue is located and interfere with the function of the organs giving rise to secondary symptoms. Other symptoms include heavy menstrual bleeding, pain during intercourse, abdominal pain, lower back pain and diarrhea during menstruation. Sometimes there are no symptoms at all.

As each person reacts differently, the degree of severity of the symptoms does not necessarily correlate with the thickness and distribution of the tissue. Having endometriosis increases the risk of uterine fibroids or breast cysts and may be accompanied by severe fatigue, chronic fatigue syndrome, or fibromyalgia (where patients' muscles ache and they feel fatigued all the time).

The only way to diagnose endometriosis is by laparoscopy, a surgical procedure in which the doctor inserts a small scope inside the pelvic cavity to look for endometrial tissues.

Treatment consists of surgical removal of the endometrial tissues growing outside the uterus together with drug therapy focusing on restoring the hormonal balance using birth control pills. Regrettably, both are not very successful long term.

More than 500,000 surgeries are performed each year for endometriosis and there is a recurrence rate of 40 percent and up for continued pain and incapacity. However, this disease often subsides with menopause when estrogen secretion is naturally reduced. It also goes away when the ovaries cease to function. Unless the absolute estrogen level in the body is reduced or estrogen dominance subsides, the return of the condition is often just a matter of time.

2. Premenstrual Syndrome

Women have long endured unsympathetic comments and attitudes towards their discomforts that occur each month like clockwork. The set of symptoms—PMS to most of us—begins soon after puberty and can last till a woman reaches menopause. Each month, she finds her body swelling. The ring on her finger gets tighter. Her breasts swell painfully. She gets tired easily. She is quick to flare up or weep. She may long for chocolate all the time—it is the body's innate response to remedy its magnesium deficiency with the magnesium in chocolate. This syndrome was first described in 1931. It is a well-established set of physical and emotional symptoms that develop after ovulation (day 14) and before the onset of the next period. The syndrome can range from a few days to two weeks.

The physical pain may be mild in some women in which case it can be relieved by an aspirin. Some less fortunate ones suffer severe and debilitating symptoms. Generally, its symptoms intensify as the menstrual period approaches. The majority of

PMS patients experience significant improvement if steps are taken to balance the body's excess estrogen.

Dr. Katherine Dalton published the first medical report on PMS in 1953. She observed that an administration of a high dose of progesterone via a rectal suppository relieved symptoms of PMS. Clearly this shows that progesterone alone can be useful in a large number of cases, and the use of synthetic estrogen for PMS may not be the right answer.

It is important to note that not all PMS symptoms are caused by progesterone deficiency and estrogen dominance. Hypothyroidism can produce similar symptoms. Stress leading to adrenal exhaustion and low adrenal reserve, commonly seen in working mothers for example, can also cause such symptoms. A diet low in fiber can cause estrogen to be re-absorbed and recycled.

> **Xenoestrogen-laced beef and poultry are now thought to contribute to PMS. Many researchers think that it may be linked to xenoestrogen exposure during the baby's life in the womb, damaging baby's follicles. The ovaries damaged in the fetus by the pollutants could result in infertility and chronic estrogen dominance decades later.**

The PMS sufferer needs to make some key dietary and behavioral adjustments. First, let us tackle the items that do the damage:

- Eliminate empty calories such as sugar, potato chips and other junk food.

- Eliminate hydrogenated fats (particularly trans-fats) such as those found in cookies and margarine.

- Reduce calcium intake and increase magnesium intake.

- Avoid caffeinated drinks like coffee and tea.

- Avoid dairy products like milk, butter and cheese.

In their place, the following will be beneficial (details are found in Part 2 of the *Adrenal Fatigue Syndrome*):

- Supplementation with natural compounds that have estrogen-clearing effects.

- Supplementation with nutrients high in omega-3 fatty acids and anti-inflammatory agents such as borage or fish oil.

- Lastly, and most importantly, the use of natural progesterone cream.

3. Fibrocystic Breast

It is a sign of the times that one of the most common reasons why women visit the gynecologist is the discovery of breast lumps. It does not take great imagination to appreciate the turmoil that such a discovery causes women. Fortunately, not all lumps are cancerous.

Typically, the following scenario would probably unfold: After a needle biopsy and scan, most patients are told that they have a benign cyst in their breast. The patients are usually reassured that the lump is not cancerous. (The next chapter is dedicated to breast cancer.) Many are sent away without any further treatment or advice. However, it is most important to alert these patients that such a lump is often the body's cry for more progesterone to counter estrogen dominance.

Breast fibrocysts often represent overgrowth of otherwise normal breast tissues. It is an early warning sign of estrogen dominance and worse symptoms to come if the hormonal situation is not remedied.

Natural progesterone cream applied directly on the breast is a good remedy. Apply 20 mg of progesterone cream from ovulation (day 12 to 14) until the day or two before the period starts. Normal breast tissue softness will return within two to three months. In addition to applying natural progesterone, supplementing with natural vitamin E (alpha d-tocopherol) and borage or evening primrose oil (omega-6) will help to reduce the inflammatory response of breast tissues. Borage oil is preferred over evening primrose oil as it is more potent.

4. Premenopausal Syndrome

Scientists have also identified a chronic condition similar to PMS, which they call premenopausal syndrome. The symptoms are similar to those of menopause but they occur often from the mid-thirties to early forties and a few years ahead of menopause. This may be due primarily to ovulation failure and the resultant lack of a corpus luteum to produce progesterone. More often than that, it is due to luteal failure. This occurs when the corpus luteum fails to produce enough progesterone in premenopausal women despite their ovulating.

In addition, there may also be stress-induced adrenal exhaustion. Chronic stress forces the adrenal gland to overwork to the point of breakdown leading to a reduction of progesterone output from the gland. Estrogen dominance sets in to produce the symptoms that patients dread. Premenopausal syndrome may include PMS, fibrocystic breasts, uterine fibroids, irregular periods and endometriosis. Apply 20 mg of progesterone cream from ovulation (day 12 to 14) until the day or two before the period starts. This can often relieve many of the symptoms.

5. Polycystic Ovary Syndrome

Polycystic ovary syndrome (PCOS) is a condition where several cysts are found on the ovaries, among other symptoms such as anovulation (lack of ovulation), menstrual abnormalities, hirsutism (excess facial hair), male pattern baldness, acne and often obesity. It is estimated that 10 to 20 percent of women today have PCOS. This figure could be even higher among young women, qualifying PCOS as an epidemic.

Under normal conditions, the hypothalamus regulates the hormone output of the ovaries and synchronizes the menstrual cycle. If some factor disrupts or stops a woman's ovulation cycle, the normal balance between the glands of her pituitary, hypothalamus and ovary will also be upset.

Patients are known to exhibit anovulation, where the follicle migrates to the surface of the ovary, but does not release the egg. The follicle clings on to its egg, eventually becomes a cyst and will not secrete progesterone even though estrogen and androgens continue to be produced. Deprived of this progesterone input, the woman's system becomes dominated by unopposed estrogen and androgen. While androgen has some antagonistic effect on estrogen, it also acts independently, leading to symptoms of androgen as well as estrogen excess. This hormonal imbalance is believed to be the main cause of PCOS.

According to Jerilyn Prior, M.D., insulin stimulates androgen receptors on the outside of the ovary. This blocks the release of the eggs from their follicles possibly accounting for the anovulation that leads to PCOS. The typical symptoms of excess hair on the face, arms and legs (hirsutism), thinning hair on the head (male pattern baldness), and acne follow from this chain of events.

The women affected by PCOS may at the same time have abnormally high insulin resistance—the so-called Syndrome X.

Insulin does not readily reduce their blood sugar level anymore. Left unchecked, it leads to Type II diabetes, unfavorable lipid patterns (high triglycerides, high bad cholesterol or LDL and low good cholesterol or HDL) and a low bone density (resulting in osteoporosis). Laboratory tests often show higher than normal circulating androgens, especially testosterone. The unbalanced male hormone accounts for the male pattern baldness, over-growth of facial hairs and aggressive behavior in such women.

Since standard tests for a woman with PCOS usually show up plenty of estrogen and since she is still having periods, there is a real danger that her doctor will assume she is still ovulating and producing enough progesterone. This is when the disorder is overlooked.

The formation of cysts in the ovaries is not fully explained by current medical theories. But there are several suspects in the line-up. One is xenoestrogens. Many environmental pollutants are believed to damage the unborn female baby's sensitive ovarian follicles. In a city setting, the exposure to pollutants is perhaps inevitable.

More and more, it has become evident that our modern lifestyle is a health risk. The stress that comes with competition in the workplace causes adrenal burnout. This is unfortunate for the lady who is short on progesterone.

The widespread use of drugs is something no one "bats an eyelid" at anymore. People simply fail to grasp the fact that Prozac® impairs our hormonal control system, including the hypothalamus. Birth control pills shut down normal ovary function. *Sometimes, the user's fertility never recovers when the pills are discontinued.*

Lack of exercise and obesity are also another probable factor. The statistics are inescapable. As expected, diet is known to have a positive link to PCOS. Apart from the amount eaten, the quality of food consumed is perhaps the more damning. The fast food controversy is raging once again, fuelled by exposés like "Supersize Me."

We realize that PCOS is the result of years of abuse to the hormonal system. Against this background, treatment strategies have to be holistic in order to produce the best and lasting results. It is recommended that PCOS patients use 15 to 20 mg of natural progesterone cream daily from day 14 to 28 of their menstrual cycle. This dosage can be adjusted accordingly if the cycle is longer or shorter than usual. The first signs of the hormones balancing out would be the disappearance of coarse facial hair and acne. However, it will take at least six months for the progesterone cream to take effect.

Once the symptoms of PCOS subside, gradually reduce the dosage of progesterone applied while monitoring for PCOS symptoms.

If the symptoms reappear, the regular dosage should be restored and progress monitored again. It would be most ideal for the patient to allow her body to return to its normal hormonal patterns. However, some women with PCOS may have too many damaged follicles and will always need some progesterone supplementation to maintain the regular cycle.

We cannot overemphasize the need to combine management of the condition with proper diet to balance the sugar level, application of natural progesterone, taking supplements to reduce estrogen metabolites, stress reduction and exercise.

6. Uterine Fibroids

An equally unnerving occurrence associated with estrogen dominance is uterine fibroids (uterine leiomyomata). They are non-cancerous tumors consisting of fibers or fibrous tissue that arise in the uterus. It is the most common tumor to grow within the female genital tract. These growths are highly sensitive to estrogen. They develop following the onset of menstruation, enlarge during pregnancy and decrease, often disappearing, after menopause when the estrogen level decreases by half. They vary in size, with the largest fibroid on record weighing over 100 pounds! It afflicts many women, especially from age 35 to 50.

One in four women in the U.S. has at least some evidence of fibroids. Discovery is usually accidental, especially when the patient seeks medical attention for heavier menstruation, irregular bleeding, and/or painful periods.

It is not uncommon for the tumor to obstruct or disrupt other organs. A recurrent example is compression on the bladder. In such cases, surgery may be required. The most commonly recommended surgery is a hysterectomy, where the uterus is removed. Many hysterectomies, however, are performed long before the patient runs out of other less radical options. The fact is that hundreds of thousands of hysterectomies are performed every year in the US alone and it is questionable whether they are necessary for the patient's well-being.

Newer and less radical procedures have emerged such as uterine artery embolization which is used to eradicate the fibroid "seed" normally present at the center of each growth. The technique is much less invasive, produces good results, and skips over the traumatic removal of the uterus. The most obvious advantage is sparing the patient the psychological distress of adjusting to the loss of an important part of her womanhood.

We appreciate by now that fibrous tissues are stimulated by estrogen. The higher the estrogen level, the faster the fibroid grows. While a fibroid in itself does not usually lead to cancer or become cancerous, it can prove troublesome to other organs. More importantly, it signals a serious underlying imbalance in the woman's reproductive and hormonal systems. Specifically, estrogen dominance appears because progesterone secretion declines. Such an imbalance does not only affect a woman's uterus but also her hormone-sensitive tissues such as the breasts, cervix, ovaries and vagina, as well.

> **Fibroids are clearly a part of the spectrum of diseases associated with estrogen dominance. Fibroids that are small can often see a size reduction when an aggressive estrogen reduction protocol is implemented. Strict adherence to an estrogen-free diet, application of natural progesterone cream, oral intake of estrogen-clearing supplements and weight reduction form the cornerstone of the fibroid reduction program.**

7. Breast Cancer

Breast cancer is a rampant epidemic, striking approximately ten percent of all adult women in the US. The greatest surge of breast cancer diagnoses is in the Western Hemisphere, from where it is now spreading globally to all industrialized countries. Among women between the ages of 18 to 54, it is the most common cause of death.

Breast cancer is usually discovered when a woman feels a painless lump in her breast. Other symptoms include an area of dimpled, creased skin on the breast, a vague discomfort in the breast, or an indentation on the nipple.

Statistics will show that the breast-cancer epidemic is also a recent phenomenon. *The finger points at the frequent use of artificial hormones in HRT.* The artificial progesterone called progestin (sold under the different trade names) is a prime suspect.

Along with the insults of other factors like xenoestrogen, a sedentary lifestyle and poor nutrition, a modern-day woman is breast cancer's sitting duck. On the bright side, study after study has shown that the majority of breast cancers in adults are not genetically linked. Only about ten percent of cases owe their origin to genetic defects. Your mother or sister's breast cancer does not necessarily mean that you need suffer the same fate.

> **It turns out that more than 80 percent of breast cancers result from estrogen dominance and can be overcome.**

In fact, with early detection, breast cancer can be cured if the body's estrogen level is brought under control as quickly as possible. It is not a coincidence that when a woman's estrogen level is cut by about half after menopause, her risk for breast cancer drops dramatically.

We shall not deal in depth with breast cancer here as the next chapter is devoted to the disease. Suffice to say that reducing estrogen aggressively is the key to preventing and treating breast cancer.

Chapter 6

Breast Cancer—The Naked Truth

Basic Breast Cancer Facts

B reast cancer is the most common female cancer in industrialized countries. It is the top cancer killer among women between the ages 45 and 50. It is a silent epidemic today, striking approximately one in every ten women. The number has gone up from one in 30 women in 1960 before hormone replacement therapy was popularized. Women taking synthetic estrogen and synthetic progesterone together had a 32 percent to 46 percent increase in their risk of breast cancer.

This statistic is based on a large pool of data from the famous Nurses' Health Study conducted at Harvard Medical School. While the body is crying out for natural progesterone to counter the estrogenic effects, the synthetic substitute only worsens the patient's problems.

It is appalling that the same FDA-approved synthetic hormonal drugs used for hormonal replacement have been documented to cause cancer and are now classified as carcinogens—substances that cause cancer.

Meanwhile, breast cancer incidences have increased 26 percent from 1980 to 1985. There were 1.2 million new cases and 500,000 deaths from breast cancer in 2000. Eighty percent of women diagnosed with breast cancer are the first in their families to get it. This tells us that the cause of the cancer does not lie in our genes only. Otherwise, the proportion of first family sufferers would be much lower.

The medical community has noted that the highest incidence of breast cancer occurs among women between their mid-thirties and mid-forties. The frequency graph rises to its peak about five years before menopause. This is a time when the level of estrogen is still high in the body whereas progesterone has already started its precipitous drop.

Studies have shown that by the time a lump is palpable in the breast, the tumor has already been there for about seven years. It would have started in the woman early in her thirties so it is not likely to be a case of estrogen deficiency. This is the time when many women in industrialized nations often stop ovulating without knowing it. As explained earlier, women suffering from anovulation have reduced progesterone in their body and face estrogen dominance.

On an optimistic note, with early detection, breast cancer is one of the more treatable of cancers. The truth remains that the average woman afflicted with breast cancer is robbed of an average of 20 years of her life.

Breast Cancer—Nature Or Nurtured?

The nature-versus-nurture debate rages on over whether cancer is inherited in one's genes or caused by the environment in which one lives. The picture has gotten clearer of late. A study published in the July 13, 2000 issue of the New England Journal of Medicine examines to what degree cancer is caused by heredity and to what extent by environmental influences.

Researchers, led by Paul Lichtenstein, Ph.D., from the Department of Medical Epidemiology, Karolinska Institute, Stockholm, Sweden, carried out investigations into tumors, including stomach, breast and lung cancers. Both studies concluded that the environment was the more influential contributor to cancer. It is estimated that more than 80 percent of breast cancers are caused by environmental and lifestyle factors. Continuous exposure to estrogen and xenoestrogen over time is the most common known risk factor for breast cancer after ionizing radiation (see section on merits of mammography in the next chapter).

In another study, a massive survey was conducted among identical twins to assess if cancer was caused by genetic factors. It looked at the incidence of breast cancer among identical twins, which naturally have 100 percent the same genes. If statistics show that both twins have the same risk, then genetic factors would seem inescapable. The results, however, reveal only a low correlation between heredity and cancer: For all types of cancer, the probability of twins getting the same disease is only about 10 percent. The researchers also noted that the rate is only slightly higher for breast, colon and prostate cancers —about 14 to 30 percent. These results published in the *New England Journal of Medicine* give us comfort that the majority—70 to 85 percent—of cancer cases are caused by factors other than heredity.

Another study lends further support for this conclusion. The researchers found that adopted children whose adoptive parents died of cancer have five times the normal risk of getting the same disease. This fact leads us to believe that something in their environment, be it their home, lifestyle or diet, plays a greater role than heredity.

Yet other studies have also noted that cancer victims are in the state they are in because of the way they live, what they have been exposed to in their lives and particularly during their early childhood. We can cite the study conducted at the London School of Hygiene and Tropical Medicine. The results tell us that cancer linked to hormonal factors is actually attributable to the patient's early childhood environment. They concluded that fraternal twins (who share at most 50 percent of their genes) have more hormonal cancers than identical twins.

Another factor suspected of causing cancer is the present day diet. With growing affluence, we are consuming more meat and with that, more animal fat. It has been established that fat intake has possible links to breast cancer along with colon and prostate cancers. Fat tissues also tend to accumulate many biochemical contaminants. Research findings from Canada and Denmark have pointed out that women with high levels of toxic residues have higher risks of getting breast cancer. Tragically, they also have the poorest prognoses.

Furthermore, Dr. Tony Zheng and his team from Yale University also found that women who enjoyed eating plenty of well-cooked red meat during the three years before diagnosis had three to four times more breast cancers than those who consumed less. The link has been traced to heterocyclic amines, a compound found in well-cooked meat which is known to damage healthy genes. Meat also contains other known cancer-causing factors: the fat-seeking organochlorines and plastic contaminants from food packaging. This conclusion is supported by another report from Columbia University who reported that high levels of cancer-causing compounds, called polycylic aromatic hydrocarbons are directly bound up in the genetic code (the DNA) of those with breast cancer.

We again stress that up to 80 percent of breast cancers are attributable to an unhealthy lifestyle and hormonal imbalance. This means that you can avoid the majority of cancers by simply adjusting your lifestyle. You have a choice.

Kinds of Breast Cancer

In the effort to understand and conquer the disease, researchers have categorized breast cancers according to how and where they grow. Some grow slowly, while others are much more aggressive. One category of breast cancer is confined entirely within a milk duct with no cancerous cells invading the tissues outside the growth or tumor. It is termed *ductal carcinoma in situ* (DCIS). Another category affects the fatty or connective tissues alone and is termed *lobular carcinoma in situ* (LCIS).

With the advent of the mammogram, it has become much easier to detect and diagnose DCIS which show up as small calcifications (hard tissue a few mm in diameter). On the other hand, LCIS does not form calcified lumps and, consequently, is more difficult to detect and recognize. Note that the size of the lumps is no indication of how virulent it will be. The statistics show that DCIS can be present in up to 92 percent of breast-cancer patients aged 30 to 39 compared to 43 percent of patients aged 40 to 49.

This means that lobular cancer occurs mostly in pre-menopausal women who often go on to develop invasive cancer although the malignancy might take up to 40 years to develop. Because of its low virulence, many oncologists do not recommend any intervention. They describe LCIS as atypical hyperplasia (meaning abnormal changes found in cells not necessarily cancerous) with a high propensity of breast cancer. On the flipside, once the ductal or lobular cells become malignant, they give the worst prognosis as their cancerous cells can spread very quickly. In general, 90 percent of breast cancers start in the milk ducts and 10 percent in the fatty tissues of the breast.

Estrogen and Cancer

This section explains in a very simplified way how estrogen, the feel-good hormone, is linked with cancer.

It is important to understand that estrogen in our body comes in three main forms—estrone (E1), estradiol (E2) and estriol (E3). Our body makes the three estrogens in the approximate ratio 10 percent E1, 10 percent E2 and 80 percent E3. The E1 and E2 are potent estrogens. They relieve symptoms of hot flashes but also promote cell growth and can lead to cancer if unchecked. By contrast, E3 is the weakest of the three forms but acts to prevent cancer. It is being used, especially in Europe, to treat breast cancer.

The risk of cancer, therefore, has to be considered carefully when it comes to any hormone replacement therapy. As always, balancing these components is critical.

Unopposed estrogen, principally estradiol (E2), is a known cause of breast cancer. This is well documented by numerous scientific studies including a seven-year research on 240,000 pre- and postmenopausal women. After adjusting for other risk factors, it concluded that using estrogen replacement therapy for six to eight years gave the subjects a 40 percent higher risk of ovarian tumors. The women who used estrogen drugs for eleven or more years had a startling 70 percent higher risk of dying of ovarian cancer.

In addition, studies also show that estradiol (E2) stimulates breast cells to form lumps in the breast. Some of these are benign or non-malignant hyperplasia. In addition, experiments have shown that estradiol stimulates and activates the cancer gene, Bcl-2, leading to cancer cell proliferation. Progesterone, on the other hand, activates the so-called p53 gene. This gene governs the detoxification system and also signals when the old cells should die. Thus, it prevents uncontrolled growth of tissues into cancers. So progesterone is important as a regulator of cell death (apoptosis) blocking the Bcl-2 gene's carcinogenic effect.

It has become increasingly clear that estrone (E1) and estradiol (E2) stimulate breast cancer while progesterone has the opposing effect. For the sake of simplicity, the use of the word estrogen is commonly taken to refer to a combination of E1, E2 and E3, with E1 and E2 forming the major proportion.

Risk Factors

Before we became aware of estrogen's role in causing cancer, doctors identified certain traits that seemed to be linked to cancer. However, we have now realized that almost all the risk factors associated with breast cancer are linked at least indirectly to estrogen dominance. We will now consider the common risk factors.

Age

Women in the age group 35 to 45 have the highest incidence of initial stage breast cancer. This age range coincides with the period of between five and fifteen years before menopause. It is a time when a woman's estrogen level is still high, while the progesterone in her system has begun to drop rapidly. After menopause, the woman's risk for breast cancer drops considerably.

Early Menarche or Late Menopause

Menarche [pronounced 'man-ark'] is the age at which a woman experiences her first period or menstruation. Unusually early menarche or overly late menopause seems to increase breast-cancer risk for women. The probable reason is that it increases the woman's lifetime exposure to estrogen. The more menstrual cycles you have, the more estrogen will be circulating in your body during your lifetime.

Heredity

After much research and debate, the consensus is that about ten percent of all breast cancers can be attributed to genetic factors passed from generation to generation. With the available DNA testing tools, the genetic predisposition to this cancer can now be detected before any breast lump is found. We have said that by the time the lump is discovered, it might have been festering for many years. As such, this is one case where surgical removal of the precancerous breast (or prophylactic mastectomy) should be considered, controversial as it may sound. Those who inherit the breast-cancer gene face a probability greater than 80 percent of getting the disease.

Pregnancy

Women who bear children before age 24 have five times less risk of breast cancer compared to women who have children after age 30.

This is seen to be the protective effect of the high progesterone level in their system during pregnancy and the lactation period. Child-bearing gives their body a holiday from estrogen dominance so to speak. Do note, however, that interrupted pregnancy (miscarriages and abortions) do not offer the same protection and may, in fact, increase the risk of breast cancer. Their risk is greater than for women who have never conceived.

Removal of Ovaries

Women whose ovaries are removed prior to age 40 have a lower risk of breast cancer. This is likely due to the reduced level of estrogen in their body. A main supply has been cut. However, estradiol has its beneficial roles and without enough of it in their system, these women will have a higher risk of suffering heart disease, arthritis and osteoporosis in later life. Such is the delicately balanced world of our hormones.

Oral Contraceptives

Girls under 18 who use oral contraceptives have three times the average woman's risk of having breast cancer. The younger a woman begins using oral contraceptives, the higher the risk. This is likely due to the synthetic progesterone used in the pills blocking the beneficial effect of natural progesterone in the body. Interestingly, women older than age 20 who have taken the pill for more than 10 years have only a slightly higher risk of breast cancer.

Hormone Replacement Therapy

There is little doubt that synthetic hormone replacement therapy practiced since the 1960s is a strong causative factor of breast cancer.

The cancer is often discovered one to three years after the woman starts on HRT. Dr. K.J. Chang and his co-workers have demonstrated in laboratory studies that estradiol increases breast cell proliferation by 230 percent! On the other hand, progesterone decreases it by more than 400 percent. When progesterone is combined with estradiol, the researchers were able to maintain a normal cell multiplication rate. The message that comes through is that unopposed estrogen should not be prescribed if breast cancer prevention is a top priority.

Obesity

You will recall that being overweight is linked to estrogen dominance of which ovarian fibroids is a symptom. To add to their woes, obese women also have a higher risk of finding fibrous growths in their breasts that can turn cancerous. In the same way, it is probably due to the presence of more free radicals and estrogen conveniently hoarded by their ample adipose tissues.

One estimate attributes up to 16 percent of postmenopausal breast cancers to obesity. Those who have gained more than 25 pounds compared to their lowest weight in adult life have up to 70 percent higher risk of breast cancer. The good news is that any sustained weight loss during premenopausal adult years will decrease breast cancer risk by 20 percent. Looking good is of course the icing on the cake.

Alcohol Consumption

Those who take more than one drink of alcohol per day also have a higher risk. This agrees with the observation that Western societies see more cases of breast cancer than societies where alcohol is not as commonly consumed by women. The fact that alcohol is a toxin is not properly accepted in Western culture. Long-term drinking puts a great strain on the liver to eliminate this drug from our system. A worn-out liver will lose its efficiency and the resulting increase in estrogen metabolites in the body are thought to be a contributing factor to breast cancer.

Insulin Resistance

A person develops a resistance to insulin mainly because of the lack of exercise and consuming too much food high in sugar. The ills associated with obesity often cause the insulin to lose its effectiveness on the sugar circulating in one's blood. Concurrently, the excess insulin also stimulates the ovaries to produce androgen. The situation is made worse when insulin resistance occurs at the same time as menopause, because insulin resistance contributes to an ever-rising estrogen level.

PCOS

In the foregoing chapters we described the causes of polycystic ovary syndrome (PCOS). It is a chain of events that cause an excess of estrogen in the woman's system. These contributory causes form cysts in the ovaries and the patient simultaneously ceases to ovulate as well. Cysts form in the ovary with PCOS as a consequence. The higher estrogen level and insulin resistance associated with PCOS is a significant risk factor for breast cancer.

Melatonin

This hormone, primarily functioning as Nature's sleeping pill, also regulates the female hormonal cycle. A high melatonin level reduces ovarian production of estrogen and increases progesterone production. The enhanced progesterone-to-estrogen ratio protects the body against breast cancer. Conversely, low levels of melatonin have been associated with increased risks of breast cancer. Air stewardesses, for example, commonly suffer low levels of melatonin. They have twice the incidence of breast cancer compared to women from other walks of life. Another piece of evidence is that blind people have an even lower incidence. Melatonin production is increased in total darkness and during sleep. Data show that blind people have a higher melatonin level than sighted people. Air stewardesses tend to have a lower melatonin level because of frequent sleep and body clock disruption from flying, especially over long hauls.

The reader should note that sub-clinical, low grade infections such as chronic viral infections can also lead to reduced melatonin production which can be a trigger for breast cancer.

Hypothyroidism

When a woman's thyroid system malfunctions, it may predispose her to breast cancer. With the thyroid hormone suppressed, there is a concurrent lowering of her sex hormone binding globulin (SHBG). This SHBG normally serves to bind tightly to estradiol and keep it from entering cells to cause mischief. Among women, hypothyroidism most commonly occurs during the perimenopausal years. This is a time when estrogen dominance creates a cycle of lowered thyroid function, decreased SHBG and a further increase in the levels of estrogen. It is not surprising, then, that natural progesterone therapy often restores normal thyroid activity.

Xenoestrogen

There is little doubt that environmental estrogen-like compounds are carcinogenic when it comes to breast cancer. These xenoestrogens can damage the ovaries and further upset the hormonal imbalance. They also suppress the immune system so that it fails to eliminate cancer cells. On top of that, they stimulate breast ductal cells to proliferate and turn cancerous.

Environmental Pollutants

Polychlorinated biphenyls (PCBs) are a class of chemicals with a variety of industrial and commercial applications. However, due to their persistent toxic effect on human health, PCBs have been banned in the US and Canada for two decades. Traces of the chemicals stubbornly linger in the environment and easily infiltrate the food chain, accumulating particularly in fatty foods.

Over the last two decades, scientists had suspected a link between PCBs and an increased incidence of breast cancer. Studies were carried out to show the correlation between the levels of PCBs detected in the system with the occurrence of the disease. The findings were inconclusive. Researchers later looked into the cancer-causing effects of 14 individual PCBs instead. This time around, they noted that high levels of two specific PCBs, PCB 118 and PCB 156, showed a 60 to 80 percent correlation with breast cancer! The link was more evident in premenopausal women. Based on a comparison between a group of 314 breast cancer patients and 523 healthy women, the study was reported in the *American Journal of Epidemiology* April 1, 2002;155:629-635.

It also found that women with high levels of a combination of three PCBs that resemble the cancer-causing chemical dioxin—PCBs 105, 118 and 156—were twice as likely to develop breast cancer. These chemicals are called mono-ortho PCBs. Again, this risk was higher in premenopausal women. It brings up the question: Does estrogen act in concert with these mono-ortho PCBs in causing breast cancer?

Stress

Stress is a silent killer in a number of ways. Causing breast cancer is one of the less well-known ones. The body under stress responds by secreting the antistress hormone cortisol. Chronic stress causes an over-production of cortisol and eventually leads to adrenal fatigue. Progesterone normally secreted by the adrenal gland is reduced in times of prolonged stress, leading to pro-longed estrogen dominance.

Studies have shown that women with breast cancer were slightly more likely to have experienced stress episodes like divorce, death of a loved one or loss of employment within two years before their breast cancer diagnosis.

However, highly significant information showed up when researchers compared women who had "intimate emotional support" as they went through their acutely stressful situations, with women who had none. Those without support had nearly ten times the rate of breast cancer compared to those who rated themselves as having good emotional support.

Mammogram

The mammogram has been touted by some to be a highly effective breast cancer prevention tool. But not all scientists agree. In Sept 2002, The Annals of Internal Medicine published the result of the longest and largest running study of mammograms ever undertaken. This is the Canadian Breast Screening Study, where over 50,000 women were tracked for 11 to 16 years. It observed those who had mammograms done and those who did not. The results showed that although more breast cancers were detected in the mammography group, there were no differences in the end in how many women died of breast cancer in each group. Simply put, mammograms do not save lives in women age 40 to 49. As a matter of fact, there is an ongoing debate on whether mammography is actually contributing to breast cancer deaths and triggering breast cancer proliferation.

The rule of thumb seems to be: Do not expose yourself excessively to radiation and compression of breast tissue that occur during a mammogram. It is sufficient for every

woman to do a careful monthly self-breast examination. If she finds a suspicious lump or dimple, then it is an indication to go for a mammogram for confirmation of her suspicion. If mammogram is necessary, take melatonin 10-30 mg one day prior to the procedure to offset any negative radiological effect of the mammogram.

Geography and Race

Women in less developed countries suffer fewer breast cancer cases than their sisters from industrialized communities. This is consistent with our belief throughout about the ills women face living in a modern society. Study after study have shown women in developed countries having a higher incidence of breast cancer. Asians on the whole, regardless of country, have a lower rate. It is very telling that among Asians who move to North American, the incidence of cancer has been found to match that of North Americans within two generations. Caucasian women in the US have the highest mortality rate from breast cancer worldwide—89 per 100,000 women. This fact is put down to social and cultural factors. Among women, this group is most likely to have early menarche, to be overweight, to use contraceptive pills, delay child-bearing till later than 24 years of age, face chronic workplace stress and live in an environment polluted by petrochemicals and other xenoestrogens.

Summary

Less than ten percent of all breast cancers are genetically linked. The rest are related to lifestyle (stress, diet and obesity) and environmental factors (xenoestrogen and environmental pollutants). Underlying this gamut of risk factors is the common denominator estrogen dominance. The root problem remains the same—an excess of estrogen without adequate progesterone to moderate it. The excess estrogen encourages the cells of the reproductive organs to grow out of control into cancerous tumors.

While normal tissue can withstand external assaults from time to time, chronic excess of estrogen or its undesirable metabolites are invitations for the tissues to go bad. Premenstrual syndrome (PMS), premenopausal syndrome, menopausal syndrome, endometriosis, fibroids, ovarian, prostate and breast cancer are all merely symptoms of the underlying cause—estrogen dominance.

The key to reducing the level of estrogen in our body is the thrust of the next part of this book.

Part 2
THE SOLUTION

Estrogen Reduction Protocol

Realistically, there is no way for us to avoid exposure to environmental estrogen. All of us suffer from estrogen dominance in one way or another. There simply is too much of it around— in plastics, car exhaust, meat, soaps, carpets, furniture and paneling. You may have no inkling that your on-and-off sinus problems, headaches, dry eyes, asthma, and cold hands and feet are attributable to xenoestrogens. In the long haul, exposure to xenoestrogens can cause more problems than just arthritis and gall bladder disease.

This part of the book is devoted to methods of avoiding the ravages of excess estrogen. The solution to estrogen dominance is actually very simple in concept.

There are three general approaches:

1. Increase your progesterone level with natural progesterone to counter the estrogen load (Chapter 7, *Natural Progesterone*).

2. Reduce your estrogen load internally through enhancement of liver function and conversion of bad estrogen metabolites into good ones (Chapters 8, *Detoxification*, and 9, *Your Diet*).

3. Reduce your external estrogen uptake through dietary and lifestyle changes (Chapter 10, *Lifestyle*).

With the above three-prong approach, estrogen dominance can often be effectively overcome.

Chapter 7

Natural Progesterone

Progesterone—Reining In Your Estrogen

While we are learning about the things that can go wrong with hormones, we must appreciate that our natural hormonal (or endocrine) system is an ingenious and very sensitive control mechanism. However, it goes awry when its natural balance is upset because of how and where we live. Estrogen in itself is not bad for us, as long as it does not dominate the other hormones that keep our body in good working order.

What we need to re-establish control over excess estrogen is natural progesterone. Even if you have only mild symptoms of estrogen dominance, natural progesterone is still valuable for its cancer prevention properties. It helps to reduce the risk of ovarian, endometrial and breast cancers.

Recall that the problem lies in the imbalance between two potent hormones estrogen and progesterone. Our priority is then to restore the balance. This will involve a whole series of actions, not simply adjusting the levels of estrogen and progesterone alone. In fact, those who have estrogen dominance and adrenal fatigue will find it difficult to restore estrogen balance without first attending to adrenal gland function.

For that matter, metabolic issues such as the imbalance in blood sugar and insulin levels are strong deterrents to any effective hormonal balancing program. There are cases when specific measures to normalize the progesterone and estrogen might not even be necessary if metabolic and adrenal equilibrium is optimized. Once the adrenal gland is working properly and the body is responding appropriately to insulin secretion again, some patients naturally regain their estrogen-progesterone balance.

The straightforward goal is to reduce the level of estrogen while increasing the level of progesterone circulating in the bloodstream. The progesterone supplement may be applied as a cream (termed topical supplementation), taken orally, or given as an injection. The physiological dose required by the body is in the range of 20 to 30 mg per day. Once the adrenal secretions are optimized, this often brings dramatic relief from PMS and premenopausal as well as menopausal symptoms.

While estrogen is known as the feel-good hormone, its counterpart, progesterone, is not well acknowledged for the part that it plays in our regulatory system. It is definitely a very versatile hormone that maintains our physical and mental health while keeping cancer at bay.

Reproductive health

We saw earlier how progesterone acts to foster our reproductive health. It ensures that a woman menstruates normally each month. Also, without an adequate level of this hormone, a woman will have difficulty conceiving and seeing her baby through to full term. In line with these roles, progesterone also promotes sex drive or libido.

Energy

It facilitates thyroid action that controls a person's energy level. Part of this action involves controlling the level of oxygen available in the blood. It in turn influences the secretion of insulin that regulates the amount of sugar in the blood. We know what excess sugar in the blood can lead to—diabetes.

Fat conversion

In a related role, it acts as a fat-burner, converting fat in the body to energy. With waning progesterone output in our twilight years, we tend to put on a lot of fat. Surprise!

Bone-building

It is also a hormone that has bone-building properties in its ability to help stimulate a type of cell called the osteoblast. Osteoblast is the precursor of the hard substance that is our bone. In other words, it is very important to bone- building. It prevents osteoporosis by increasing bone density and strengthening brittle bones in the patients.

Natural diuretic

A diuretic is a substance that makes us lose body water by inducing urination. Without it, our body tends to retain water. Together with accumulated fat tissues, water retention results in the feeling of being bloated.

Normalizing zinc and copper levels

While it regulates the amount of water in our body, progesterone also maintains optimum levels of the two important minerals, zinc and copper, in our body.

Anti-cancer action

Cancer, as we have said, is a disease in which the cells in a certain part of the body keeps multiplying, growing, and encroaching on their neighboring organs. By opposing the growth-promoting effect of estrogen, progesterone keeps cancers in check. In particular, it acts against endometrial and breast cancers and also protects against fibrocystic breasts.

Sense of well-being

Progesterone is a natural antidepressant. Together with all the energy-promoting, libido-increasing properties, it generates a sense of well-being we all need to get up each morning and look forward to another meaningful day.

Natural vs. Synthetic Progesterone

We now proceed with a word of caution. Progesterone supplements are very potent, as all hormones are. Next, remember that, for commercial purposes, pharmaceutical companies often prefer to manufacture their drugs from convenient raw materials in a laboratory. This makes perfect business sense. However, drug companies often produce synthetic drugs that only approximate the amount of biochemical a patient actually needs. Progesterone is one such example.

A synthetic hormone called progestin, which closely resembles progesterone is produced and sold under various trade names. It is not identical to natural progesterone—not the real McCoy, so to speak, and is metabolized in the liver into byproducts that are toxic if present in excess. The built-up metabolites can severely interfere with the body's own natural progesterone. In fact, synthetic progesterone is so powerful that it strongly monopolizes the body's progesterone receptors and renders natural progesterone ineffective most of the time. The displaced natural hormone is unable to stimulate the p53 gene to secrete the chemical messenger that tells tumors to stop growing. This results in an increased risk of cancer.

There are also other functional differences between natural and synthetic progesterone. Natural progesterone, you may recall, is the hormone that favors conception and pregnancy. Contrast this with the contraceptive properties of synthetic progesterone contained in a pill combined with estrogen. More directly, progestins have been successful and commonly used in a program to terminate pregnancy.

Pity all the women put on synthetic progesterone during menopause because they feel bloated due to water retention. Other undesirable side effects of the synthetic drug include increased risk of birth defects if taken during the first four months of pregnancy, exacerbated hormone imbalance leading to mood swings, abnormal menstrual flow, acne, hirsutism (excess facial and body hair), masculinization, increased incidence of blood clots, nausea, insomnia and depression. It is not to be used if the person has thrombophlebitis (veins swollen by a blood clot usually in the leg) or liver dysfunction. It is suspected of causing malignancy of the breast and the genitals. One of its metabolites has an anesthetic effect. Users are often lethargic, depressed, and do not respond to antidepressants such as Prozac.

Fortunately enough, natural progesterone is commonly available. It is derived from wild yam and has the same chemical structure and properties as those of progesterone secreted naturally in our body. The progesterone is produced by extracting diosgenin from wild yams and then converting this active agent into natural progesterone in the laboratory. The wild yam-derived progesterone is labeled natural or bio-identical progesterone. It is this supplement that should be applied.

Today, we have access to many of these bio-identical plant-based hormones, either through prescription or over the counter. The body recognizes them as its own hormone.

It is important to note, however, that simply taking wild yam as such will not balance your hormones as the body has no mechanism to convert wild yam into progesterone. So do not be misled by products that are advertised as containing wild yam extract. The way to make sure that progesterone is present and not simply wild yam extract is to look for the "USP progesterone" on the label. USP stands for United States Pharmacopoeia, which is the international standard for purity.

Side Effects Of Natural Progesterone

There are no known side effects if natural progesterone is applied in physiological amounts under normal conditions. This means 20 to 30 mg a day for women and 6 to 10 mg a day for men (men are also affected by estrogen dominance, a major contributor to prostate cancer). It is, therefore, very safe. But as with most pharmaceutical substances, too much progesterone is actually counterproductive. A chronically high dose of progesterone over many months eventually causes progesterone receptors to turn off, reducing the supplement's effectiveness. Some possible side effects of over-dosage include:

- An anesthetic and intoxicating effect such as slight sleepiness. Excess progesterone down-regulates estrogen receptors whereas the brain's response to estrogen is needed for the production of serotonin (the hormone that regulates our mood). This is solved by simply reducing the dosage until the sleepiness goes away.

- Some women report paradoxical estrogen dominance symptoms for the first week or two after starting natural progesterone. This is normally caused by a resensitization of estrogen receptors by the progesterone. The symptoms generally resolve themselves spontaneously within a few weeks. Patients may feel anxious, have difficulty sleeping and retain water. Hot flushes may also be experienced. Their weight may increase with their appetite.

- The edema (water retention) is likely to be caused by excess conversion of progesterone to deoxycortisone, a mineralcorticoid made in the adrenal glands that causes water retention.

- Candida is a yeast in our digestive system which normally helps to curb other bacteria. It is controlled by other good bacteria in our gut and our body's defenses like white blood cells. Excessive application of progesterone can inhibit anticandida white blood cells, which can lead to a proliferation of an invasive growth of candida. This results in bloating and gas. Systemic candidiasis can be treated with a grain-free diet for two weeks and temporary discontinuation of natural progesterone, followed by gradual building up doses of progesterone cream.

Routes of Progesterone Delivery

As we have said before, natural progesterone can be supplemented orally, topically or by injection. Taking it orally is less efficient as less of it is absorbed, so a higher (pharmacological) dose is required. Although injection is more effective, it can cause irritation at the injection site. To achieve the most effective physiological dose, applying the cream is best.

Progesterone is easily absorbed by the skin. It is five to seven times more effective in reaching the bloodstream than oral forms of progesterone. Quantitatively, 100-200 mg of oral progesterone is needed to obtain the equivalent benefit of 20-30 mg of progesterone cream (doctors sometimes use the term trans-dermal progesterone).

For the best stabilization of progesterone absorption and effectiveness, apply the cream in two divided doses, once in the morning and once at bedtime. Progesterone vaginal gel is sold under the trade name Crinone. This is a good way of delivering progesterone to contiguous areas. For fibroids, polyps, or an overgrowth of endometrial tissues, this is the preferred method of delivery. The gel is applied to the "G spot," an area located at the top of the vagina. While absorption is good anywhere in the vagina, the fastest absorption occurs here. A concentration of 10 percent of the gel is commonly used. A quarter teaspoon contains about a gram of the bio-identical progesterone. It is also available in concentrations of 4 to 8 percent.

Those who find it more convenient can consider the oral form in a capsule called Prometrium. This is a proprietary product developed in Europe from yams. It is approved by the FDA for use in combination with estrogen drugs to prevent endometrial hyperplasia (overgrowth of cells in the endometrium) in menopausal women. It is available in 100 to 300 mg potencies in daily dosages.

Fortunately, most women do not need such high doses. It is also far more advantageous to have hormonal intake twice a day to protect the body throughout the 24 hours. Ask your doctor and your pharmacist to compound a non-proprietary formula for you, at a lower dosage, in the form of natural progesterone capsules. These are available in potencies from 25 to 100 mg. They are prepared by a so-called micronization process. Take them with meals to enhance absorption. Start with 100 mg at night and 50 mg during the day (to avoid drowsiness).

Oral progesterone is also available in the form of sublingual drops to be applied under the tongue. The most common concentration available is 50 mg per eight drops. Sublingual drops are useful for PMS and conditions where frequent adjustments are needed. Use a maximum of five to six drops at a time. If you take more, there is a tendency to swallow some of it which decreases the rate of absorption. Repeat the drops after a brief rest if more is needed.

Delivery Systems of Topical Progesterone

To effect maximum absorption to pass the skin barrier, natural progesterone is carried in an oil/water emulsion that contains the same fatty acid composition as the skin. On the other hand, mineral oils will prevent the progesterone from being absorbed into the skin.

The cream should contain 400 to 600 mg of natural progesterone per ounce. Each one-half teaspoon application would supply a minimum of 26 mg of progesterone (women usually produce about 20 mg of progesterone daily under normal circumstances). To simplify matters, some of the pharmaceutical companies package the cream with a metered dispensing bottle. One pumpful of it delivers about 20 mg of progesterone. To get the physiological dose, women commonly apply one pumpful a day (20 mg) in two divided doses of half a pump each, while men apply half a pumpful a day (10 mg).

Without such a dispensing bottle, some reckoning is needed. Assuming that the absorption rate of the cream is 50 percent, we need to apply a cream with 480 mg of progesterone in total in order to absorb the 240 mg required. The recommended regime is to find a cream with 480 mg progesterone per ounce. Apply 1/8 to 1⁄2 teaspoon of the cream per day over two to three weeks.

The consumer should read the label carefully to apply the right dosage. Surveys have shown that many commercial progesterone creams contain less than 15 mg of progesterone per ounce. In fact, some of these creams contain as little as 2 mg of progesterone per ounce. Clearly not all formulas are created equal.

Low vs. High Dose Progesterone Cream

Progesterone cream concentrations come in a range from 1.5 to 10 percent. Some medical experts advocate the use of a low-dose cream. The renowned Dr. John Lee felt that an excessively high-dose (10 percent) progesterone cream is quickly metabolized in the liver and some of the metabolites may have an anesthetic effect on the brain, causing lethargy and depression. Also, progesterone is rapidly absorbed from the skin and there will not be a steady, sustained release of progesterone into the bloodstream. Since progesterone has a half-life of only five minutes once it is in the blood, a sudden rush of progesterone very soon loses its effectiveness.

Other doctors, notably gynecologist Dr. Uzzi Reiss, feel that a higher-dose cream works better if patients have fibroids. At 10 percent concentration, each gram contains 100 mg of progesterone. To deliver the normal physiological dose of 20 mg a day, much less is needed.

Laboratory Measurement

To be sure that your progesterone level is optimum, you may seek the services of an analytical laboratory. Salivary or blood serum hormonal testing will provide a measure of your current level of free hormone in the body and assess the amount of natural progesterone that you need. A note of caution. Do not be over dependent on laboratory testing. A significant number of people do not fall within the laboratory reference range and can still be estrogen dominant. Conversely, many may be considered normal by laboratory test and yet have symptoms consistent with estrogen dominance. Finding a health professional who is experienced is far more important than relying on laboratory tests, whether it be saliva or serum.

The nature of the body's absorption and transportation systems is such that the level of the progesterone delivered through the skin will rise much faster in the saliva than it will in the bloodstream. The level can be measured within three to four hours in the saliva. Serum tests, however, are carried out after months of proper application of the progesterone cream. In general, it takes about three to four months for the progesterone in the body fat to reach a physiologically steady level for those who have reached menopause, and about one to two months for those who are premenopausal.

Serum levels measure the total progesterone available which is much higher than the biologically active portion. Normal premenopausal women will show a level of 7 to28 ng/ml (nanograms per ml. A nanogram is a billionth of a gram.) during midcycle (the luteal phase). In contrast, normal postmenopausal women will show a level of 0.03 to 0.3 ng/ml without treatment. After three months of topical progesterone, it should rise to 3 to 4 ng/ml, an increase of ten- to a hundredfold. This level is sufficient to correct osteoporosis in postmenopausal women. The serum level of progesterone is best tested around day 19 to 22 in a 28 day cycle, when its level is highest.

It is easy to see why saliva testing is gaining popularity over serum testing. It is easier to administer, the results are obtained faster and it is an accurate measure of the free progesterone level in the system. The salivary level of topically applied natural progesterone goes up within three to four hours and is washed off by eight hours. It takes the blood level months to stabilize if one were to take serum progesterone levels.

How To Apply Progesterone Cream

Progesterone is best absorbed where the skin is relatively thin and well supplied with capillary blood flow. Areas such as your face, neck, upper chest, inner arms and thighs are good areas. Spread the cream out to as big an area as possible for maximum absorption and allow all the time you can afford for the application. Therefore, bedtime is best if you are applying it once a day. Twice-a-day application is better but it may be too troublesome for most. Rotate to different areas to avoid saturation and desensitization in any one particular site.

Here is a sample, twice-a-day rotational application protocol:

Day 1 morning: Apply to the right side of the back of the neck.

Day 1 before bed: Apply to the left side of the back of the neck.

Day 2 morning: Apply to the right wrist area above the palm.

Day 2 before bed: Apply to the left wrist area above the palm.

Day 3 morning: Apply to the underside of the right upper arm.

Day 3 before bed: Apply to the underside of the left upper arm.

Repeat this cycle from day 4 onwards. In other words, day 4 will be the same as day 1, day 5 will be the same as day 2, and so forth.

From a practical standpoint, the best gauge for the ideal dose should not be any laboratory test alone. As an indication, it is also important to rely on the relief of symptoms—how you feel with the application. The right dose is the dose that works.

Paying for Your Doctor's Ignorance

Many physicians still believe that menopause is caused by the fall in estrogen levels only. These same physicians are also unaware that the progesterone level falls earlier than that of estrogen as a woman approaches the change of life. There are those doctors who are unaware that a patient can be within the normal range in one hormone and yet have hormonal imbalance relative to other hormones. For them, it means prescribing more estrogen – causing a vicious cycle of the patient's symptoms. This misguided opinion needs to be put right. The fact is that estrogen only falls by about 50 % in this transition. The majority of postmenopausal women continue to make estrogen in the fat cells. During the aging process, the amount of sex hormone binding globulin (SHBG) rises. This effectively binds to estrogen, making free estrogen (the one that really counts) less available.

Other doctors who do not keep abreast of developments think that the synthetic progesterone called progestin is a good substitute for natural progesterone. By prescribing synthetic estrogen with synthetic progesterone, these physicians think that the patients are protected. This is a fallacy. Natural progesterone behaves very differently. If a reminder is necessary, the reader is advised to revisit the section above about the risks of using synthetic progesterone if a reminder is necessary.

Starting on Progesterone

Over sixty percent of all women in their perimenopausal phase of life and almost all women in menopause are deficient in progesterone. They are the population that is at greatest risk of the symptoms and illnesses associated with estrogen dominance.

For them, natural progesterone replacement is the route to go, especially if estrogen is being supplemented. Success stories abound. Patients have expressed satisfaction with their progesterone supplementation and their restored hormonal balance. Some have lost as much as four pounds of retained water. Their PMS have disappeared overnight. Engorged and tender breasts have regained their size and comfort. Patients have become more relaxed and have better sleep. Energy levels have risen dramatically.

First Things First—A Thorough Check-Up

Before any progesterone cream is applied, get a physical and gynecological checkup, clinical breast examination and pap smear. Make sure that your adrenalin and insulin levels are corrected if correction is necessary. A pelvic ultrasound is also helpful to measure thickness of the uterine lining. The following are general recommendations that may need to be modified for the patient's specific circumstances:

Women In Perimenopause and Still Ovulating

Most women in perimenopause should consider progesterone supplementation. From age 35 onwards, progesterone production in the body begins its decline. By the time a woman reaches perimenopause, the amount of progesterone circulating in her system would be drastically low. Generally, supplementation is required only two weeks out of a month, from day 12 to 25.

If your estrogen secretion is still appreciable, expect full periods—in other words, heavy bleeding. In this situation, more progesterone can safely be used to offset the excess estrogen.

If your estrogen is low, or if you have signs of estrogen deficiency, progesterone may prevent you from having another period. We must emphasize that progesterone can only be applied two weeks out of a month. Continuous application each day can lead to frequent light bleeding.

Four Common Occurrences

Adjusting the amount of natural progesterone needed during perimenopause is tricky as the body is undergoing rapid change. While on progesterone, the following four occurrences are commonly encountered:

- If you have occasional spotting, there is no need for alarm. You may safely continue with the supplementation.

- If you spot or get your period before the end of the two weeks on progesterone, you need a higher dosage provided that there are no side effects. If you have maximized your dose and the problem still persists, consult your physician to rule out fibroids or other uterine growths.

- If you experience heavy flow of blood, discontinue the supplementation. Consider this the first day of a new cycle and resume the hormone two weeks later.

- If your period does not come within a week of completing the first cycle of supplementation, consider the last day of supplementation as day 1 of a new cycle and resume applying progesterone on day 12.

Those on No Hormonal Supplementation

- Count the day the period begins as the first day.

- Apply 20 mg (one pumpful in a metered pump dispenser when properly dosed) of natural progesterone every day from day 12 to 25. Those with a longer cycle may have to use it from day 10 to day 28.

- Begin the cream after ovulation that usually occurs about 10 to 12 days after your period begins.

- If bleeding starts before day 26, stop the progesterone and start counting up to day 12, and start again.

Those on Synthetic Progesterone

Gradually taper off the synthetic progesterone or progestin (whatever the trade name) and replace it with natural progesterone a little at a time over a three- to six-month period. Reduce your daily pill intake to every other day and then increase the interval further.

Those on Synthetic Estrogen and Progestin Combination

Combinations of synthetic estrogen and progestin are commonly prescribed. It would be obvious to you now that both these synthetic hormones have undesirable effects on your system. Replace your prescriptions with natural progesterone gradually. Recall that a synthetic estrogen will prevent natural progesterone from working since it binds to receptor sites more strongly than real progesterone does. Furthermore, synthetic estrogen is not excreted as efficiently as natural progesterone is.

You should apply 15 to 20 mg natural progesterone at bedtime. Also, since Prempro® comes with synthetic estrogen, ask your doctor instead for bio-identical estrogen and natural progesterone instead. If synthetic estrogen is absolutely needed as a stopgap, then ask for a prescription of Premarin® (a conjugated estrogen) 0.625 mg and take half the dose (that is 0.3125 mg) a day. Reduce the Premarin® dose by half every two to three months while staying on natural progesterone.

Perimenopausal Women Still Menstruating With Menopausal Symptoms or PMS

You will find that a natural progesterone cream can relieve menopausal symptoms and prevent osteoporosis.

Count the day your period begins as the first day. Apply 20 mg of natural progesterone from day 7 to day 27. If your period begins early, stop using the cream when you start your menstruation.

If oral progesterone is used, take 25 to 200 mg daily in divided doses.

Women in Menopause

These women face problems caused by falling levels of both estrogen and progesterone although estrogen is still probably more dominant. The regime for preventing or reversing their osteoporosis and relieving menopausal symptoms will depend on their other hormonal supplementation habits. The recommended regime must balance out the negative side effects of the excess estrogen, decrease water retention, promote relaxation and better sleep, and aid the body's defense system against cancer.

Those Not on Estrogen Replacement Therapy

Choose a convenient day to begin, such as the first day of the month. Apply 20 mg of natural progesterone daily in two divided doses from day 1 to 25. Let the body rest without supplementation for the rest of the month.

If a woman has not been producing progesterone for a number of years, her body-fat store of progesterone will probably be very low. In this case, double up on the application for the first two months and return to the normal physiological dose thereafter. Do this by increasing the dosage every few days to a total of 40 mg a day.

As we have said, go by how you feel to determine if you have reached an optimum dosage. You may have some symptoms of estrogen dominance like hot flushes as the estrogen receptors are being resensitized.

For those on oral progesterone: Take two 50 mg strength capsules half an hour before bedtime. Next morning, take one 50 mg strength capsule. This can be increased by 50 mg each night until restful sleep is achieved, or when side effects of paradoxical reaction such as water retention, foggy thinking, or depression are relieved.

Some women can tolerate up to 300 mg a day, while others cannot. For some, breaking up the dosage into four times a day works better than twice a day.

If three months of applying progesterone cream, eating a proper diet, and taking nutritional supplementation of magnesium and vitamin B6 do not relieve the symptoms, then low-dose natural estrogen may be considered. Applying 2.5 mg of natural tri-estrogen cream (10 percent estrone, 10 percent estradiol and 80 percent estriol) provides the equivalent action of 0.625 conjugated estrogens such as Premarin®.

Those on Estrogen Replacement Therapy

Reduce the dosage of the estrogen supplement to half when starting on natural progesterone. Otherwise, the woman would

110

likely experience symptoms of estrogen dominance during the first two months of progesterone. Every two to three months, reduce the estrogen supplement again by half. Estrogen and natural progesterone can be used together during a three-week cycle each month, leaving a rest period of seven days without either hormone. The estrogen dose should be low enough that monthly bleeding does not occur but high enough to prevent vaginal dryness or hot flushes.

Those Taking an Estrogen and Progestin Combination

Stop using the synthetic progesterone immediately when starting on natural progesterone cream. Estrogen should be tapered off slowly. These patients typically complain of being overweight and not having the ability of shedding the unwanted pounds. They have water retention and swollen breasts. Their doctors often put them on tranquilizers or sleeping pills to settle their anxiety. It is not unusual for these patients to come home from the doctor with a bag full of drugs including Xanax®, Valium®, Halcion®, or Tylenol®.

If unrelieved by progesterone cream alone, low-dose natural estriol may be added for three weeks out of the month in cases of menopausal symptoms such as vaginal dryness and hot flushes. Alternatively, the use of low-dose estradiol or tri-estrogen cream (natural estrogen cream by prescription) can be applied.

Premenopausal Women with Hysterectomy or Ovaries Removed

Apply 20 mg of progesterone for the first 25 days of the calendar month and rest from day 26 to the end of the month.

If the ovaries have been removed, careful attention should be paid also to estrogen replacement therapy (only bio-identical supplements). In this case, symptoms of testosterone deficiency should also be expected. Androgen replacement with 0.15 mg of a supplement cream can be very effective. Under no circumstance should estrogen replacement be carried out without opposing progesterone. It will worsen your condition.

Menstrual Migraine

Apply 20 mg of progesterone cream during the ten days before your period (day 16 to 26). Apply a small amount, like 5 mg, every three to four hours when you sense the aura (the side effect that affects sensory functions like speech) coming or until symptoms cease.

Flagging Libido

Both men and women suffer a loss of the sex urge when their sex hormone levels fall. It is a fallacy that this is the inevitable consequence of aging. Progesterone and testosterone are both important factors in upkeeping libido. Testosterone is the much more potent solution but natural progesterone can be tried at 20 mg a day for women and 6 mg a day for men.

Hair Loss

When progesterone level drops due to ovarian follicle failure and a lack of ovulation, the body responds by increasing the synthesis of androstenedione, an adrenal cortical steroid. This has some androgenic properties, resulting in male pattern hair loss.

Natural progesterone supplement of 20 mg a day for six months may be helpful to reduce the androstenedione level, so that, over time, normal hair growth will resume.

Hypothyroidism

The thyroid hormone and estrogen have opposing actions. Protocols that oppose estrogen tend to improve the symptoms of cold hands and feet, skin problems and respiratory infection indicative of low thyroid function. These symptoms of hypothyroidism, occurring in patients with unopposed estrogen or estrogen dominance, often diminish when progesterone is supplemented.

Women who have normal thyroid function and are on progesterone but still have the symptoms, should have their adrenal function investigated by a doctor. If needed, supplemental natural cortisol may be required for short term use if adrenal fatigue is diagnosed.

Other Specific Uses Osteoporosis:

It is proven that there is significant bone loss during the 10 to 15 years before menopause, despite an ample supply of estrogen in our body during this period. For more than half a century, estrogen was given routinely with the promise that it would cure osteoporosis. Today, it has been well established that estrogen replacement therapy does reduce fractures from osteoporosis by 50 percent.

Purely in terms of osteoporosis prevention, however, this approach is not recommended. Osteoporosis is a complex process that we have yet to fully understand. The role played by estrogen is controversial at best. Let us see why:

While we now know that estrogen inhibits the bone-destroying osteoclast cells, estrogen cannot rebuild bone. Another type of cell called osteoblasts are the solder of the bone building process. It is progesterone that is required to stimulate the osteoblasts to form the hard bone matter. As we have said, the estrogen levels in the premenopausal years are considerable though reduced.

During this same period, however, most women experience a drastic reduction of progesterone in their body. Clearly estrogen replacement alone is not the answer.

Supplementing with natural progesterone has proved useful in preventing and reversing osteoporosis. In other words, progesterone, not estrogen, is the key to healthy bones.

In the 1990 July issue of the *International Clinical Nutrition Review* on the effectiveness of natural progesterone, Dr. John Lee administered natural progesterone cream to healthy 35-years-olds. In the first 6 to 12 months, subjects had a 10 percent increase in bone density instead of an annual decrease of 3 to 5 percent. It showed that reversal of osteoporosis is indeed possible through the use of natural progesterone alone. Some patients had up to twenty to 20 - 25 percent increase within a year. The beneficial effect of progesterone is not affected by age but the initial bone density. Those with the lowest bone density scores showed the most improvements. It is apparent that progesterone can help, no matter how far the bones have degenerated.

Dr. Lee's study also showed that the addition of estrogen to natural progesterone did not make the progesterone more effective. His subjects used estriol only to relieve menopausal symptoms and not to treat.

Dr. Lee's findings were confirmed by Dr. Jerilynn Prior of the University of British Columbia.

Recently researchers have discovered some types of plant materials that mimic the effects of estrogen. Compounds called phytoestrogen, contained in the plants, act as weak estrogens. While consumption of phytoestrogen has been linked to reduced symptoms of menopause, it is unclear if osteoporosis is prevented.

When progesterone and estrogen supplementation do not increase bone density in women with osteoporosis, it is usually because they have low androgen (DHEA and testosterone) or high cortisol levels.

Apply 20 mg daily in two divided doses from day 1 to day 25 of the menstrual cycle. The patient's baseline bone mineral density (BMD)—an index of bone strength—should be measured. Repeat the test after a year. If the BDM is increased, the dose can be reduced by half. If BMD does not increase, other factors such as exercise, diet and optimization of nutrition should be undertaken together with a full medical checkup to identify other underlying causes.

PMS

PMS is usually accompanied by higher levels of cortisol and stress. We have said that this secretion by the adrenal gland is the body's response to stress. The excess cortisol competes with your progesterone hormone for the same progesterone receptor site, and also reduces progesterone production. You will, therefore, need more progesterone to stave off the ill effects.

Apply 20 to 40 mg a day for the first month, from day 12 to day 25. Some patients have found it quite beneficial to apply the cream in a crescendo pattern, starting with a small dab at night and gradually increasing to two dabs per morning and night, and finishing off with bigger dabs up to three times a day in the final three days.

Dosage can be reduced once the symptoms improve. There are normally multiple causes of PMS, so in addition to progesterone cream, other hormonal boosters may be required. It is also good to take anti-inflammatory supplements like borage oil.

If you suffer premenstrual migraine headaches, apply 20 mg of progesterone cream during the ten days before the period begins. Be alert to the aura—the temporary speech or other sensory disruptions—that usually precedes these migraine attacks. You can apply a small glob (1/4 to 1/2 teaspoon) every three to four hours till symptoms subside.

To overcome hot flushes, apply a small dab to the inside of the wrist at the onset of the symptoms.

Irritable Bowel Syndrome

Commonly known by its initials, IBS refers to a set of disorders like indigestion, constipation and diarrhea that do not have physiological or biochemical cause.

> **Many women, we are happy to note, have reported reduced IBS symptoms a few months after starting on natural progesterone. Progesterone has a calming effect on the immune system and the bowels. However, the exact mechanism of action is not fully known.**

Uterine Cramps

This can be prevalent during the menstrual period. Relief can often be found by applying a physiological dose of natural progesterone cream directly above the pubic area at onset of the cramps.

Polycystic Ovary Syndrome

Patients with PCOS produce very little progesterone. To overcome the symptoms, apply 20 mg of progesterone cream from day 14 to day 28 of the menstrual cycle. Adjust accordingly for longer or shorter cycles. As the hormonal balance is regained, facial hair and acne, two commonly associated symptoms, will disappear.

Infertility and Miscarriage

According to Dr. John Lee, one of the chief causes of early-term miscarriage is the failure of the body to increase progesterone production sufficiently during the first weeks after fertilization.

> **Women who have difficulty conceiving or who may be at risk of such an early pregnancy loss may wish to discuss beginning natural progesterone supplementation with their physician.**

Postpartum Depression

Postpartum depression is a serious medical condition that can be devastating to both the mother and the child. While the exact cause is still not known, many researchers suspect that the drastic fall in progesterone immediately after childbirth may play an important role. While in hospitals, patients can be treated with an injection of 200 mg of progesterone daily. Estrogen should also be supplemented while in the hospital, often with an estrogen patch. When the patient goes home, this combination should be replaced with natural progesterone cream 10 to 20 mg twice a day plus Tri-Est® gel or 2.5 mg capsule twice a day.

Breast Cancer Prevention

Breast cancer occurs most often during estrogen dominance. Dr. Graham Colditz of Harvard Medical School postulated that unopposed estrogen is responsible for 30 percent of breast cancer. A preventive protocol is application of low-dose natural progesterone cream (12 to 15 mg per day). Your doctor will probably prescribe applying it over 24 to 25 days a month if you are at risk.

Breast Cancer Management

Progesterone supplementation should be maintained for life with all breast cancer patients, before, during and after surgery. According to Dr. Lee, there is no contraindication with concurrent use of other anti-estrogen drugs like Tamoxifen®. In plain words, this means that there is no ill effect in using natural progesterone if you are taking Tamoxifen® as chemotherapy. Generally speaking, a higher dose of the cream is needed compared to healthy menopausal women without eliciting any side effects.

Uterine Fibroids

Use 20 mg of progesterone cream from day 12 to day 25 for small fibroids. An ultrasound test can be obtained initially to determine the size of the fibroid. Repeat the scan after three to six months of use to see the improvement. A 10 to 15 percent reduction in size is generally attainable if the fibroid is small. The bigger the fibroid size at the time of starting progesterone, the lower the chance of it reducing in size but, generally, you can at least expect the size not to increase. This is the effect when progesterone speeds up the clearance of estrogen from your system.

If the strategy works, continue this treatment until menopause. At menopause, the progesterone application can be reduced. Fibroids normally shrink after menopause as the estrogen level decreases. If the fibroid is already large (tangerine size), more progesterone may not help but instead may contribute to its growth.

This paradoxical reaction may be due to the series of responses to the degeneration and cell death within the large growth. It sets up an inflammatory response with white blood cells invading the dead tissues as part of their "clean up" job. In this process, estrogen is created within the fibroid itself and growth factors are secreted which can be stimulated by progesterone. In such a case, monitor the progress carefully with ultrasound. Surgical removal may be necessary if the growth continues unabated.

Endometriosis

Apply 20 mg of natural progesterone cream starting from day 8 and continuing to day 25 of a usual 28-day cycle. The dosage may be adjusted to match the relief of symptoms. It may take six months or more before the full benefit of the regime is realized. The dosage may be increased if no effect is experienced after two months. As the desired result is obtained, the dosage can be reduced. Do note that too much progesterone can cause drowsiness and other minor side effects earlier discussed.

Breast Fibrocysts

Breast fibrocysts are an overgrowth of normal breast tissue. Apply 20 mg of progesterone cream from ovulation (day 12 to day 14) until a day or two before the period starts. Breast tissue normally softens and will return to its normal state within three to four months. Also take 400 IU of vitamin E at bedtime, 600 mg of magnesium and 50 mg of vitamin B6 a day. Refrain from coffee and reduce your sugar and fat intake. Once the symptoms subside, the dosage can be adjusted downwards.

Summary

Using natural progesterone cream is a cornerstone of the estrogen reduction protocol. Not only will natural progesterone counterbalance estrogen, it is a hormone that has many other benefits as well, from bone building to mood enhancement. Proper application is the key and using low doses of 20 mg per metered pump of natural progesterone cream is the easiest method (you can add more later).

Chapter 8

Detoxification

Any compound that has a detrimental effect on our cell function or structure is said to be toxic and toxins are substances that poison our system. We become aware of fast-acting toxins almost immediately. But there are those that accumulate slowly in our system without noticeable harm immediately. They have long-term consequences that patients bear in the course of time. Now, thanks to consumer education, we have become more aware of their presence and danger.

Regrettably, toxins come with the technological advances that humankind has achieved. The machines and conveniences we enjoy in urban life bring with them polluting industrial chemicals and byproducts that wreck our body's defense system. It is inconceivable that an industrial city can get rid of the heavy metals that escape from factories into our environment. Nor can we envisage living without using insecticides sprays for the home, preservatives in our food and pesticides for our food crops.

Some of our social habits, if uncontrolled, expose us to more danger. Of these habits, cigarette smoking is the most prevalent. The disease agent in tobacco smoke is tar but some additives have also been implicated. Non-smokers are now acknowledged to suffer from breathing secondary smoke from their environment.

The other very prevalent practice is having that social drink. However, research has shown that one alcoholic drink a day, in the case of postmenopausal women, can increase estrogen in the body by as much as 16 to 20 percent and two to three drinks a day can increase it by up to 30 percent. In premenopausal women, two to three alcoholic drinks a day reduce levels of progesterone while increasing levels of estrogen.

This may be due to the toxic effect of alcohol causing reduced clearance of estrogen in the liver. The excess estrogen not metabolized by the liver will continue to circulate and exert its undesirable effect on the body. Caffeine from coffee also has been proven to increase estrogen level significantly.

There are other seemingly innocent sources of toxins. Aluminum from your cookware, soda cans and antacids; mercury from dental fillings and fish caught in polluted waters; additives in our food; and the household chemicals that mimic our hormones can behave like estrogen, leading to estrogenic effect.

The worse news is that many toxins tend to accumulate in our body. Being fat-soluble, especially if they are petroleum-based, most of these toxins and all steroidal hormones such as estrogen, progesterone and testosterone incorporate themselves into the fatty tissues of the body where they stay for years. So, even if our daily exposure to them might seem negligibly low, the symptoms will hit us after long years of toxin buildup in our organs or body fat. The organs affected include the brain, breasts and endocrine glands such as the thyroid and adrenals. Once entrenched, it is difficult for the body to eliminate. The toxic effect, if not normalized, can last for decades.

Resulting symptoms include memory impairment, foggy thinking and hormonal imbalance resulting in adrenal gland dysfunction, hypothyroidism, PMS, breast pain and infertility. That is not all. Such toxins as xenoestrogens, including pesticides and petrochemicals, are all carcinogenic. They contribute to or are strongly associated with the rising tide of cancers.

This chapter offers us a way out of this trap. Detoxification can rid your body of the accumulated toxins. While many different detoxification approaches have been defined, they differ in their actions and purpose. Some detoxification programs only affect the bowels. Others may cleanse the liver or blood. Yet others may aid the kidneys or the skin in their functions.

The key detoxification organ when it comes to hormonal balance is the liver. It is here that the hormones are broken down into metabolites to be excreted out of the body. An optimized liver will help clear estrogen from the body, while an under-performing liver will only allow the body to become toxic by accumulating unmetabolized hormones in the body.

Approaches that must be considered in the detoxification process are nutrition, supplementation, water, exercise, rest, sunshine and fresh air. By combining these detoxification programs into a total estrogen clearing program, one can effectively restore the healthy hormone balance state.

Detoxification Centers of the Body

Nature has provided us with a very sophisticated system of defense against illnesses. The majority of us take this for granted when we enjoy good health. The fact remains that the system is vulnerable to abuse whether we do it deliberately or not. If the abuse is discovered, timely action will help to rehabilitate a body that has been weakened by toxins. An understanding of how our defense system works will be useful to our appreciation of how we should keep it in working order.

To deal with substances that poison us, the body has in place several centers of detoxification.

The Skin

Our skin acts like smart wrapping paper for our precious insides. It is our first line of defense against harmful environmental agents. However, it is not totally impenetrable to every harm. We have seen how transdermal application can be an effective means of introducing progesterone into our system. Equally, some toxic chemicals can be absorbed through the skin as well.

However, to a certain extent, the skin acts as a cleansing organ for us. Skin extracts toxic wastes from the blood and excretes them through our sweat glands and dead skin. In this way, toxins such as DDT, heavy metals and our own urea are eliminated when we perspire or shed old skin.

The Liver

This is a very versatile organ. One of its chief functions is to cleanse our blood of toxins. It filters blood to get rid of bacteria and other non-living chemical toxins. The bile secreted by our gall bladder passes through the liver where cholesterol is filtered out from the bile before it is allowed to digest oily foods in our intestines. The liver also helps break down hemoglobin in old red blood cells and excess proteins in our body into harmless byproducts to be excreted. Alcohol beyond a certain concentration is harmful to our system and is broken down in the liver too.

All drugs prescribed and all fat-soluble hormones, including estrogen and progesterone, are processed in the cells of the liver in an effort to render them safe for our body. It employs enzymes (chemicals that speed up the breakdown) inside the liver cells. All these activities have a profound effect on regulating and balancing our hormonal and immunal defense systems.

The Alimentary Canal

The alimentary canal is the biological term for our gut in which food is digested, which means taken apart and absorbed. The inside of our gut is lined with a membrane that secretes mucus. While it smoothens the passage of food through the canal, the mucus also removes toxins produced by bowel bacteria. Other harmful substances not digested will be expelled from the canal as excrement while fat-soluble toxins are excreted in the bile that finds its way through the gastrointestinal tract and out of the body through bowel movement.

The Kidneys

Much of the water-soluble byproducts of detoxification in the liver is carried away in the blood to the kidney. The delicate arrangement of filters in the kidneys then separates toxins and waste byproducts (urea is produced when the liver breaks down excess proteins) from the beneficial nutrients that we need. The unwanted and harmful substances are eliminated as part of our urine or sweat.

The Liver Detoxification Pathways

As far as hormonal balancing goes, no organ is more important to us than the liver. Here, hormones are broken down and cleared from the body to maintain the perfect balance required for our well-being.

The liver acts on individual xenoestrogens as they are detected. It utilizes enzymes to try and break down these fake hormones, resulting in byproducts called metabolites. These enzymes either work alone or in tandem with another agent. Thus, the liver has two mechanisms designed to help detoxify the body. They are called Phase 1 and Phase 2 detoxification pathways.

Phase 1 Detoxification Pathway

In Phase 1 detoxification, enzymes present in the liver cells help convert toxins into metabolites through a series of chemical reactions such as oxidation, reduction and hydrolysis.

One example of the Phase 1 pathway involves the cytochrome P-450 enzyme. Toxins are rendered harmless in this process and excreted through the kidneys. At the same time, free radicals are often produced which, if present in excessive amounts, can damage the liver cells. Fortunately, the body has a built-in protection mechanism. Antioxidants, such as vitamin C and E and natural carotenoids, can neutralize these free radicals and reduce the damage caused.

If the body lacks the necessary antioxidants and the toxin exposure is too high, the toxic chemicals escape detoxification by the liver. Some of them may be converted from relatively harmless substances into carcinogens.

It spells trouble when our body is laden with pollutants from our environment or toxins that we take in as a social activity or even as part of our medication. Too much of pesticides, alcohol or prescribed drugs can disrupt the P-450 enzyme pathway by causing overactivity, when this pathway is put into overdrive. Caffeine, saturated fats, trans-fat, paint fumes, car exhaust, cigarette smoke and barbiturates can bring on this overactivity. As a result, the level of free radicals rises dangerously inside the body. We need a wide variety of antioxidants to fight free radical overload and enhance Phase 1 detoxification.

Phase 2 Detoxification Pathway

Phase 2 detoxification by liver cells involves a process called *conjugation.* The liver enzyme requires another agent to help it get the job done. It may work together with a cysteine, glutathione, glucuronide, sulfur or glycine molecule to overcome the toxic drug or chemical which has entered the body. Once conjugated, the metabolite compound is neutralized and rendered less harmful to the body. The drugs, toxins and hormones are converted into substances that are eventually excreted from the body via our bodily fluids such as bile or urine.

It stands to reason that any substance that harms the conjugation agents will undermine Phase 2 detoxification. One example of such a substance is the enzyme beta-glucuronidase which digests the agent glucuronide. There is hope for arresting this subversive agent. Studies have shown that calcium d-glucurate, a natural ingredient found in certain vegetables and fruits, can inhibit beta-glucuronidase activity, resulting in increased elimination of toxins from the liver. Supplements of calcium d-glucurate will enhance the glucuronidation pathway critical in the conjugation process. In addition, methionine, folic acid, taurine and N- acetyl-cysteine are very useful synergistic nutrients that will help detoxification along this pathway.

Estrogen Metabolism

All estrogen (E1, E2 and E3) and progesterone are broken down in the liver. This is especially important for estradiol (E2). The liver has several pathways to convert E2 to metabolites that have a wide variety of biological activities.

Estrone (E1) is the second most potent estrogen in circulation. It is easily converted back and forth from E2 through enzymatic reactions. Both E1 and E2 are metabolized by a process called hydroxylation.

Some of the hydroxylated products are converted into estriol (E3), while others are further broken down and excreted from the body. E3 is further conjugated in the liver and excreted in the urine.

Premenopausal women normally produce several hundred micrograms of estradiol every day. Some of this estradiol finds its way to binding to the nuclei of many different tissues, resulting in genetic transcription as well as cellular division. This is intended to replace old cells in the tissue that die.

While the production of estrogen is going on, a similar amount of estradiol is removed from the body, primarily in the liver. This ongoing production and destruction process results in a constant level of estradiol in our body. It is part of the process of keeping our bodies in equilibrium.

Since the metabolites are estrogen derivatives, they all possess estrogenic properties in varying degrees. The degree of the hydroxylation provides an indication of the metabolite's estrogenic potency.

The metabolic pathways are complicated in their design. One metabolite is often converted into another but the reverse conversion can also happen. There may be multiple conversion pathways for the breakdown of some metabolites as well. This is the body's way of making sure that, even if one system fails, there is a back-up system in place.

Metabolites such as 2-hydroxyestrone or 2-hydroxyestradiol are considered good estrogens. They are also derived from hydroxylation of estrone and are the most prevalent metabolite of estradiol and estrone. These good estrogens are not as prevalent in people who are obese and in women whose diets are high in animal fat. These good estrogens can be increased by exercising consistently and moderately, following a diet high in protein and low in fat, and consuming food containing indol-3-carbinol (I3C) such as cabbage and broccoli. In addition to being good estrogens, both 2-hydroxyestrone and 2-hydroxyestradiol have been found to be powerful antioxidants and can protect the lipid proxidation process by circulating iron molecules.

Another metabolite of estrone is called the 16 alpha-hydroxyestrone. This is called the genotoxic form of estrogen, a bad estrogen. It has been shown to be more potent than estradiol. Due to its ability to combine with estrogen receptors and transform the nuclei that synthesize DNA, it increases the risk of breast cancer significantly. For this reason, it is also called the transforming estrogen. Another bad metabolite is 4-hydroxyestrone. This is a free radical generator and its role as a "bad estrogen" is still under intense investigation.

It should be clear that, just as there are good and bad cholesterols, we have good and bad estrogens as well. Being a potent antioxidant that has anticancer properties, 2-hydroxyestrone is considered good. Both 4-hydroxyestrone as well as 16-alpha–hydroxyestrone are considered bad. At high levels, they are thought to be important indicators of cancer risk. Ideally, the ratio of 2-hydroxyestrone to 16-alpha-hydroxyestrone as detected and measured in the urine should be 2.0 or higher.

Studies have shown that 73 percent of breast cancer patients have a ratio below 2.0. In other words, their 2-hydroxyestrone level is low in comparison with 16-alpha- hydroxyestrone. Other studies have also shown that women, 35 years and older, with breast cancer, have 2-hydroxyestrone to 16-alpha–hydroxyestrone ratios lower than control groups. The bottom one-third of the women studied (those with the lowest ratios) showed a 30 percent greater incidence of cancer than the higher two-thirds.

On the basis of the studies, it is now accepted that the ratio of 2-hydroxyestrone to 16-alpha-hydroxyestrone is a significant indicator of breast cancer risk in women.

Fortunately, both metabolite levels can be measured conveniently in the urine making it a straightforward test.

Consider the following factors that affect estrogen metabolite levels:

1. Obesity reduces the level of 2-hydroxyestrone in the urine and, therefore, reduces the ratio of 2-hydroxyestrone to 16-alpha-hydroxyestrone. This suggests that it is a breast cancer risk to be obese—another reason to shed those pounds.

The Asian diet, which is high in soy products and low in animal fat, has the effect of increasing the level of 2-hydroxyestrone while reducing the other estrogens, particularly 16-alpha-hydroxyestrone. Therefore, in theory, it has a beneficial effect as far as increasing the good estrogen in the body goes.

In breast cancer cases, however, this has to be taken with a grain of salt. While 2-hydroxyestrone is considered a good estrogen, it, nevertheless, falls within the estrogen family and has properties consistent with estrogen's generic nature as a pro-growth hormone.

For breast cancer patients, especially those who have tested positive for estrogen dominance, the phytoestrogen and isoflavones found in soy products should be avoided.

2. Cruciferous vegetables cabbage, broccoli, turnip and mustard, kale, Brussels sprouts, cauliflower and collard—are a rich source of indolylmethyl glucosinolate (glucodrassicin) that, on enzyme action, releases indole-3-carbinol (I3C). This I3C is then broken down by the strong acid in the stomach to form di-indolylmethane (DIM). Both I3C and DIM are known to be anticancerous. Some studies have shown that I3C can block the normal proliferation of cancer cells exposed to estradiol metabolite in the form of 16-alpha-hydroxyestrone.

3. Smoking increases the level of 16-alpha-hydroxyestrone but reduces estrogen over-all; the net effect is that smoking decreases the ratio of 2-hydroxyestrone to 16-alpha-hydroxyestrone. This is a danger signal for

breast cancer. It is interesting to note that the evidence linking cigarette smoking with an increase in 16-alpha-hydroxyestrone formation has a mechanism similar to how I3C and DIM reduce the risk of hormone-dependent tumors.

Do You Need Detoxification?

Few of us have the good fortune of living in a pristine environment free of toxins, pollutants and xenoestrogens. The air that we breathe is polluted with xenoestrogen, the water that we drink is full of chlorine, the clothing we wear is made of artificial fabrics full of toxic chemicals, the lotions and shampoos that we use all contain xenoestrogenic solvents. Once these chemicals are inside our body, we can never fully eliminate them unless we undergo an intensive detoxification process regularly.

Signs that you need detoxification are clear as day, even though you may not recognize their underlying toxic origin. You need to detoxify your system:

- If you have estrogen dominance even without symptoms of it.
- If you have unexplained headaches or back pain.
- If you have joint pain or arthritis.
- If your memory is failing.
- If you are depressed or lack energy.
- If you have unexplained weight gain.
- If you have brittle nails and hair.
- If you have abnormal body odor, a coated tongue or bad breath.
- If you have psoriasis.
- If you have frequent allergy attacks.

- If you have a history of heavy alcohol use.

- If you have a history of using a steroidal hormone, natural or synthetic.

- If you have a history of exposure to cleaning solvents, pesticides, diuretics, and drugs.

Benefits of Detoxification

The first and most important benefit of a course of detoxification is getting rid of your system's overload of estrogen. You can then look forward to life without the pain of estrogen dominance. Simultaneous with that, the other hormones especially the thyroid and adrenals, will also be restored and your growth hormone enhanced. The protocol helps to cleanse your digestive system of accumulated waste and harmful bacteria. Your stomach size is restored when you change your eating habits. Dependency on habit-forming items like sugar, caffeine, nicotine, alcohol and drugs will be a thing of the past. Your detoxification mechanism is immediately improved through the restoration of your liver, kidneys and skin. All these will stimulate your immune system. To crown it off, all your mental faculties will also be rejuvenated.

A regular detoxification program will help prevent chronic opportunistic diseases such as cancer, diabetes, chronic fatigue and arthritis. We cannot recommend it too strongly to you.

Detoxification Protocol

There are three stages to a detoxification program.

1. Preparation

Before detoxification can proceed, the body and especially the liver must be optimized. Toxins that are stored in the body tissues must be removed and metabolized by the liver and eliminated from the body. *If the liver function is not optimized before the program gets underway, the organ will be overwhelmed by the overload of the toxins swirling through the system.* As a result, you may suffer symptoms of fever, vomiting, nausea, nervousness and confusion. People have been known to be seriously sick because of the sudden, massive assault of toxins dislodged from the body because of a mishandled detoxification program.

A whole regimen of nutritional supplements should be considered:

A. Antioxidants

Antioxidants such as vitamins A, E and especially C are essential for detoxification as they help the cells to neutralize free radicals that cause cell mutation and damage. This is critical during the Phase 1 detoxification process in the liver where free radicals are released.

The vitamins should be taken together—as a cocktail—in optimum amounts because each vitamin is unique and works on a particular part of the body. For example, both vitamins A and E are fat-soluble and are found in our fat tissues. They are particularly effective in preventing the oxidation of cell membranes, which are made up of phospholipids, a fatty substance.

On the other hand, vitamin C is water-soluble and fights free radicals in blood plasma. It interacts with vitamin E to regenerate each other as well. Vitamin C is especially vital in any detoxification program, as the body needs it for energy to process and eliminate wastes.

B. Methionine

Methionine is one of the essential amino acids needed for good health. It is a valuable nutritional compound of multiple benefits to the body. Methionine is an especially important nutrient beneficial for correcting estrogen dominance. Similarly, those who are on oral contraceptives or estrogen replacement therapy will find it to be very helpful.

One of the important functions of methionine is to supply sulfur and other compounds required by the body for normal metabolism and growth. Without an adequate supply of sulfur, our body will not be able to make and utilize a number of antioxidant nutrients. Methionine is also a methyl donor. This fragment of a molecule, with a single carbon atom tightly connected to three hydrogen atoms, called a methyl group, is vital to a wide variety of chemical and metabolic reactions inside our body. Together with choline and inositol, methionine belongs to a group of compounds called lipotropics which help the liver to process fat in the body. The body can convert methionine into cysteine, a precursor of glutathione. Because glutathione is the key Phase 2 neutralizer of toxins in the liver, this is an obvious detoxification aid.

Specifically, methionine converts the stronger and carcinogenic estradiol (E2) into estriol (E3), the good estrogen. However, the body cannot produce it and so must obtain it through diet. Meat, fish, eggs, yogurt and other dairy products are all excellent sources of methionine. Vegetarians can obtain it from whole grains, garlic, lentils and onion. Beans are a relatively poor source of this amino acid.

Most people do extract enough methionine from a balanced diet. The daily requirement varies depending on the body weight. Most doctors agree that approximately 100 to 1000 mg a day is sufficient for those who are not estrogen dominant. As a rule we do not need methionine supplementation if we are in good health. That said, strict vegetarians and anybody who follows a low protein diet should consider supplementing their supply. Your doctor may recommend methionine supplementation with a concurrent intake of taurine, cysteine and other sulfur-bearing amino acids, as well as folic acid and vitamin B6 for the best results. For estrogen dominance, the recommended dosage ranges from 500 to 4,000 mg in divided doses throughout the day. Anybody with symptoms of estrogen dominance, including breast cancer should consider this course of methionine supplementation.

Take care to avoid an excessive dosage when the patient suffers from folic acid and vitamin B6 deficiency. It can increase the conversion of methionine to homocysteine which is linked to heart disease and strokes. Such patients need supplementation of folic acid and vitamin B6 as well. Despite the cautious note, supplementation of up to 4,000 mg of methionine daily for long periods of time has not been associated with any serious side effect.

A daily dose of five grams of methionine has been linked to reduced lymph rigidity and an improvement in Parkinson's disease. In Europe, doctors use it with excellent results to treat depression, inflammation, liver diseases and certain muscle pains. Such are the properties of this very versatile supplement.

C. SAMe

S-Adenosyl-methionine (SAMe) is a metabolite of methionine with many good attributes. A daily dose of up to 1,600 mg has been used to fight hepatitis and cirrhosis, consequences of liver damage. Besides this valuable role, another major application of SAMe involves the alleviation of depression. A dose of 800 to 1,600 mg a day helps to elevate the patient's mood and provide relief for the clinically depressed. Both methionine and SAMe also have anti-inflammatory effects and are often used in combination to treat osteoarthritis. SAMe is also helpful to those who have multiple sclerosis. Its anti-inflammatory properties have also proven helpful with fibromyalgia when taken at 1 gram a day. In Britain, methionine as well as SAMe are quite frequently used in the treatment of chronic fatigue.

D. Taurine

Taurine is an important amino acid in our body. It is found mostly in our central nervous system, skeletal muscle and, in greater concentration, in our heart and brain. Our body produces it from two sulfur-containing amino acids, methionine and cysteine, in conjunction with vitamin B6.

Cysteine, like methonine, is found in egg yolk and meat and, to a lesser extent, in vegetable proteins. As expected, taurine is commonly found in animal protein but not in vegetable protein. Shellfish has an abundance of it. Vegetarians lacking dietary meat protein may have difficulty producing taurine in their bodies. They will have to be mindful about the amount of taurine they need.

Taurine keeps potassium and magnesium inside our body cells while keeping out excess sodium. In this sense, it works like a diuretic, expelling sodium with excess water. But unlike prescription diuretics, it does not act against the kidney, but improves kidney function instead.

Taurine is very useful in fighting tissue swelling and fluid accumulation. People with heart failure, liver disease, late stage ovarian cancer and congestive heart failure frequently have unwanted fluid accumulating inside their bodies. Exploiting the same property, taurine has been very successfully prescribed for people with high blood pressure. Taurine also functions to dampen the sympathetic nervous system, thereby relieving arterial spasms. Helping the blood vessels relax will also bring down the blood pressure too.

Aside from that, taurine strengthens heart muscles and maintains proper calcium balance which reduces muscle cramps. Together with CoQ10 and carnitine, taurine is able to preserve the heart's contractility and guard against the toxic threat of chemotherapeutic drugs such as adriamycin and doxorubicin. Prescribed with magnesium, taurine is also used to regulate and stabilize heart rhythm.

Taurine's diuretic property helps to prevent fluid retention during menses. However, the female hormone estradiol depresses the formation of taurine in the liver. Women who are on estrogen replacement therapy, the birth control pill, or suffering from estrogen dominance may need more taurine.

Furthermore, chemotherapy and the lack of good bacteria in the intestinal tract limit the production of taurine in the body.

Expect your doctor to prescribe one to three grams a day. The general dosage for people who have edema, high blood pressure and seizure disorders ranges from 0.5 to 4 grams a day. However, at a dosage of more than five grams a day, taurine may occasionally cause loose stool and may also slightly increase the secretion of stomach acid.

E. Fish Oil

A diet with generous amounts of fish oil increases the ratio of 2-hydroxyestrogen to 16-alpha-hydroxyestrogen. Recall that this ratio is an indicator of breast cancer risk. The higher the ratio, the better it is. This is based on observations that the consumption of fish oil inhibits the formation of human breast-cancer cells in laboratory studies.

Further analysis suggests that the beneficial effect stems from the substances EPA (eicosapentaenoic acid) and DHA (docosahexaenoic acid) found in fish oil.

Be warned that not all fish are created equal. These beneficial nutrients are found only in deep- and cold-water fish. Comparisons show that fish caught in warmer coastal waters typically have lower concentrations of EPA and DHA and a higher concentration of the inflammatory arachidonic acid (AA) compared to cold-water fishes. In addition, AA has a tendency to transform into substances that have been linked to cancer (specifically breast and prostate cancers) or that adversely affect estrogen metabolism. It has been established that EPA and DHA inhibit the conversion of AA into its toxic derivatives known collectively as ecosinoids. PGE2 (Prostaglandin E2) is the ecosinoid linked to breast and prostate cancers.

Another group, called leukotrienes, causes twitchiness or hyper-reactivity of the airways in our respiratory system and triggers off asthma attacks.

F. Calcium-d-glucarate

Calcium-d-glucarate (CGT) occurs naturally in some vegetables like bean sprouts. One of its derivatives, D-glucaro-1, 4-lactone (1,4-GL) has been found to have anticancer properties. It acts against the potent enzyme beta- glucuronidase. By inhibiting beta-glucuronidase and preventing the related harmful chemical reaction (known as glucorodination), 1,4-GL increases the detoxification of carcinogens and tumor promoters. Laboratory studies comparing CGT with a known chemo-preventive agent, 4-HPR, at various phases of cancer, showed that CGT was on par overall. In particular, during the Initiation Phase (I), Promotion Phase (P) and Initiation plus Promotion Phase (I+P), CGT reduced tumor multiplicity by 28 percent, 42 percent and 63 percent respectively as compared to 4-HPR which reduced tumor multiplicity 63 percent, 34 percent and 63 percent respectively. Better yet, the studies showed that CGT and HPR administered together worked synergistically to increase their cancer-prevention power.

A daily consumption of 100 to 300 mg of CGT is recommended for ridding the system of glucoronidating toxins.

G. Silymarin

Much research has been done on a remarkable extract of milk thistle (Silybum marianum) known as silymarin, a group of flavonoid compounds. These compounds protect the liver from damage and enhance the detoxification process.

Silymarin acts as a powerful antioxidant. It is much more effective than vitamin E and vitamin C. Experiments show that liver damage in animals due to extremely toxic chemicals such as carbon tetrachloride, amanita toxin, galactosamine and praseodymium nitrate could be protected by silymarin.

Moreover, silymarin has been shown to increase the level of glutathione by up to 35 percent. We know that glutathione is an important agent for Phase 2 detoxification. The higher the glutathione content, the greater the liver's capacity to detoxify harmful chemicals. In support of this view, human studies have shown the positive effects of silymarin in treating liver cirrhosis, chronic hepatitis, fatty infiltration of the liver and inflammation of the bile duct.

The common dosage for silymarin is 70 to 200 mg, one to three times a day.

H. Lipoic Acid

Called the universal antioxidant for its ability to dissolve readily in water as well as in fat solvent, lipoic acid increases the potency in other antioxidants. It can cross the blood-brain barrier while many other nutrients such as vitamin C cannot. One of the most beneficial effects of lipoic acid is its ability to regenerate other essential antioxidants such as vitamins C and E, coenzyme Q10 (CoQ10) and glutathione. The evidence is especially strong for the ability of lipoic acid to recycle vitamin E. This is apparently achieved directly by quenching tocopherol radicals or indirectly reducing vitamin C or increasing the levels of ubiquinol (a derivative of CoQ10) and glutathione that in turn helps to regenerate tissue levels of vitamin E.

The suggested dosage is 125 to 1,000 mg daily.

I. Quercetin

Extensively researched, this flavonoid damages only cancer cells and leaves normal cells intact. In doing so, it acts synergistically with chemotherapy agents like tamoxifen, cisplatin, adriamycin and radio therapeutic agents. It is a potent inhibitor of the enzyme aromatase and helps to control the production of estrogen by the body's glands.

By reducing the metastatic potential of cancer cells it inhibits the spread of cancer. Like reishi and maitake mushroom, it stimulates the immune system acting as a potent antioxidant and free radical scavenger and disrupts the mitotic cell cycle and genetic expression in tumor cells.

Most importantly, it is anti-angiogenesis (preventing proliferation of vessels in cancer cells) due to its ability to bind tightly to estrogen receptor sites. By rehabilitating mutant p53 genes, it enhances apoptosis (natural cell death) and arrests cancer growth. At the same time, it inhibits mutant p21 genes found in over 50 percent of colon cancers. The rogue p21 signals DNA replication in cancer cells. In addition, it increases the intracellular glutathione level. Quercetin also works well in tandem with hyperthermia treatment protocols. Similarly, vitamin C enhances the effectiveness of quercetin and vice-versa.

Food sources with quercetin include onion and apples. The suggested daily dosage is 350 mg to 4,000 mg.

J. Grape Seed Extract

In 1951, a French researcher named Dr. Jacques Masquelier patented the process of extracting proanthocyanidin oligimers (PCO) from the bark of the European coastal pine tree. The extracted proanthocyanidins, which are powerful antioxidant nutrients from the bioflavonoid family of compounds, were named Pycnogenol® (pronounced Pick-nah-geh-nol).

Nineteen years after Dr. Masquelier patented the process, PCO was also found and extracted from grape seeds. Pycnogenol®'s bioflavonoid concentration is 85 percent while that of grape seeds stands higher at 92 to 95 percent. The grape seed extract is also much cheaper.

The extracted PCO functions the same way as vitamins C and E. By scavenging free radicals, it fortifies Phase 1 of the liver detoxification pathway, resulting in an increase of estrogen clearance.

Being very soluble in water, PCO is rapidly absorbed and is distributed throughout the body within 20 minutes. Its effects last as long as 72 hours after it is taken. It works very well with other antioxidants like vitamin C, quercetin and lipoic acid; in fact, it enhances their efficacy.

PCO also arms the human body with excellent antioxidant support for a variety of body repairs. This is achieved when PCO inhibits the enzymes that breakdown collagen in our body. Collagen is the protein that gives our muscle tissues their strength and tone. So PCO makes capillaries more robust so that they do not easily rupture. This makes PCO very useful in blood-vessel related conditions like varicose veins, peripheral hemorrhage, diabetic retinopathy, high blood pressure, hardening of arteries and impaired blood flow to the brain.

Compared to other nutrients normally prescribed for the above conditions, PCO demonstrated as a threefold improvement of damaged capillaries. The results usually noted include delayed signs of aging, improved circulation as well as a stronger immune system.

PCO should be taken in addition to and not in place of established antioxidant vitamins such as C and E.

The recommended dosage is 100 to 1,000 mg a day.

Significantly higher dosages are needed for specific problems. To limit heavy menstrual flow, up to 3,000 mg a day may be required. Therapeutic effects can be seen as early as in one month of use, with menstrual flow reduced from a week to four days.

2. Cleansing

Cleansing of the body system is done internally through fasting and helping the liver metabolize toxins. It is done externally through thorough skin cleansing. Enemas can also be used but are normally reserved for cases where intense cleansing is required, as is often the case when detoxifying to treat cancer. An example is the coffee enema used in the Gerson Therapy.

A. Fasting Cleanse

The principle is to stop eating any food that might remotely add to your toxin load for a chosen period of time. Cleansing by fasting can last from one day to a week. This depends on the time available, the body's requirements, the toxic load and the patient's overall health. Masses of accumulated waste are expelled as the body rids itself of toxins. You may experience short bouts of headaches, fatigue, body odor, bad breath, diarrhea or mouth sores. However, digestion usually improves immediately, as do many organ and nerve functions.

One of the most important studies regarding fasting and detoxification appeared in the *American Journal of Industrial Medicine* in 1984. In this study, patients who had consumed food contaminated with PCBs (polychlorinated biphenyls) went on a seven- to ten-day fast. All subjects reported improvements in their health and dramatic relief after fasting.

The best way to proceed is to start slow with a three-day vegetable juice fast. Longer fasts require strict medical supervision, while shorter fasts can usually be conducted at home by oneself. It is essential to consult a physician especially if you have medical conditions, such as diabetes, that may be worsened during a fast.

Prepare for fasting on the day before by eating fresh fruits and vegetables at the last meal. During the fast, take a high potency multiple-vitamin and mineral formula to provide general support. Take 1,000 mg of vitamin C three times a day and one to two tablespoons of a fiber supplement at night before sleep. If you are particularly overloaded with toxins, supplement 70 to 210 mg of silymarin three times a day.

During a fast, the body temperature usually falls. Blood pressure, pulse and respiration rates will also drop to reflect a slowdown of the body's metabolic rate. It is, therefore, important to stay warm. More rest is encouraged to yield better results, as energy can then be directed towards healing instead of other bodily functions. A nap or two during the day is recommended. Less sleep will be needed at night since daytime activity is lower. When it comes to breaking your fast, it is important to reintroduce solid foods gradually by limiting portions. Overeating is counterproductive. It is a good idea to eat slowly and chew thoroughly. Serve the food at room temperature.

Vegetable Juice Fasting

An excellent way to good health via toxin removal is vegetable-juice fasting. Vegetable juices without their pulp are an excellent source of vitamins and minerals. The juice is preferred over the vegetable whole. One can easily drink the juice of several heads of lettuce at one go, but imagine eating the same amount of whole lettuce! Vegetable juices also contain loads of antioxidants and enzymes needed for toxin cleansing. They enhance liver function and, therefore, help the metabolism of estrogen. At the same time, they eradicate digestive problems.

From the juices, the body gets plenty of nutrients for the minimal digestive action, and valuable digestive enzymes can be preserved. Moreover, fasting on vegetable juices allows the body to have sufficient time to process these juices. Fasting gives you a sense of well-being, renewed energy, clearer thinking and a cleaner body system.

For a dietary switch, vegetable juicing is not easy. So start slowly by drinking only one or two ounces each time. Gradually increase the portion to 12 ounces. If you do it right, there should be no waves of nausea or belching.

Vegetable or Fruit Juice?

Fruits have an inherent disadvantage compared to vegetables: a high sugar content. Not only will the undesirable effects of extra sugar affect someone with hormone imbalance, but a diet of fruit juices will also raise the blood sugar for a diabetic person and create unfavorable consequences.

Using the same argument, carrots and beets are also high in sugar content even though they are vegetables. They, too, can raise the blood sugar level much like fruits do. However, their natural sweetness and other beneficial nutrients make them a good starting point until the beginner's taste buds are trained. Thereafter, they should be minimized during a fast.

We acknowledge that vegetable juices are not as pleasant-tasting as fruit juices. The beginner should just gulp down the juice. This will ensure minimal contact with the taste buds. As you get used to it, or even get to enjoy it, you may learn to sip and savor the juice.

As vegetable juicing is not a natural practice, the body will need some time to adapt. It is important to pay heed to your body's signals on which vegetable juices to consume and which types to moderate. Take some whole vegetables before, during or after the juicing. The chewing motion will stimulate gastric juice secretion and aid digestion.

The pulp, disregarding palatability, is one of the most beneficial parts of the juice. It adds bulk and fiber to your diet and helps bowel movement. Try mixing 10 percent of the pulp back into the juice and slowly increase the proportion in accordance with your tolerance. Very few people can consume all the pulp with the juice. It is quite thick and looks more like a porridge than a drink.

All vegetable juices should be consumed immediately. Vegetable juice is one of the most perishable foods. As a rule, do not keep for more than 24 hours. This makes storage very tricky as oxidation should be prevented. If you have to store the juice, put it in a glass jar with an airtight lid and fill it to the brim to minimize the air space over it. Air (remember air contains 20 percent oxygen) will oxidize and ruin the juice. Wrap the jar with aluminum foil to block decomposition by light and then store it in the refrigerator. A dark-glass jar could also be used instead. The juice should be taken out of the refrigerator 30 minutes prior to consumption, as it should ideally be drunk at room temperature.

The beginner should start with the sweeter vegetables like carrot and beet before venturing on to celery, fennel (anise) and cucumbers. These vegetables may not be the most nutritious but at least they are more tolerable and palatable than others. As you get used to the taste of green vegetable juices, progress to spinach, cabbage, bok choy, endive and lettuce. Herbs such as parsley and cilantro can also be added to juices if you fancy their aroma. The advanced juicer should enjoy collard greens, dandelion greens and mustard greens. These vegetables are quite bitter tasting but they are good for you (see section on cruciferous greens).

To make your juice more palatable, you can also add small quantities of carrots and beets as a natural sweetener. Coconut is another option to improve the taste of vegetable juices. It is also a good source of fat to balance the meal.

Beginner's Juice Recipe

Carrot, 200 grams: It is high in the antioxidant beta-carotene and full of wonder enzymes. Because of its high sugar content, it should not be overused.

Celery, 200 grams: It is high in sodium—not the artificial kind but natural sodium—that promotes tissue flexibility.

Beet root, 200 grams: Beets root nourish the liver which is one of the most important and most versatile organs in the body. If your liver is functioning well, your body is likely to be in optimal health. Again, avoid overuse because of its high sugar content.

Cabbage, 200 grams: Cabbage juice is high in vitamin C and I3C (see following section). It has the added advantages of being one of the cheaper vegetables and is available all year round.

Method

Wash the vegetables thoroughly under running water. Clean with a soft-hair brush if necessary, especially with the root vegetables. Cut into rough pieces to fit the juicer. Blend the vegetables and consume it immediately. Add more and more of the pulp filtered out by the juicer as you get used to it. The recipe is enough for one glass.

Simple 24-Hour Juice Fasting Detoxification Program

Juice fasting enables the digestive system to rest. It also speeds up the growth of new cells, which in turn promotes the healing process. A person on a juice fast should abstain from solid foods and only drink fruit and vegetable juices, water, and herbal teas throughout the day. While vegetable juices are superior to fruit juices on a day-to-day basis, fruit juices are often recommended as part of a fasting program to overcome faintness due to hypoglycemia (insufficient blood sugar). It must be stressed that short spells of hypoglycemia do no long-term harm to our health.

How frequently the juice is taken varies from person to person. For most healthy persons, once a day is plenty. For those with serious conditions, round the clock juicing once every two hours is not unusual. Frequent juicing will supply the body with adequate amounts of energy throughout the day. In addition, drink at least eight to 12 glasses of water every day during the fast. Avoid coffee, bottled, canned or frozen juices and soft drinks. Unsweetened herbal teas are acceptable.

- The night before: Eat a simple dinner with a green leafy salad. Dry brush your skin before you go to bed to open your pores for the night's cleansing eliminations. (Read more about skin cleansing below.)

- On rising: Drink one glass of juice consisting of two freshly squeezed lemons, one tablespoon of maple syrup and eight ounces of water (filtered but not distilled) at room temperature.

- Mid-morning: Take one glass of cranberry juice concentrate to promote bowel movement.

- Lunch: Drink one glass of fresh apple juice.

- Mid-afternoon: Have one cup of herbal tea unsweetened.

- Dinner: Drink one glass of papaya or pineapple juice to enhance enzyme production or another glass of apple juice.

- Before bed: Have one cup of mint tea, miso soup or hot water for relaxation.

- Next morning: Break your fast with fresh fruit and yogurt. Eat light, raw foods during the day and a simple, low-fat dinner.

- The same plan can be extended over the weekend for a three-day detoxification program.

B. Skin Cleanse

Good skin care is essential to good health as our skin is one of the most effective excretion organs. When we sweat, heavy-metal compounds are eliminated through the skin's pores. Research has shown that our sweat glands can perform detoxification just as effectively as one or both of our kidneys. However, in the process, the skin will build up a toxic load. It is, thus, vital to perform skin cleansing from time to time to keep the skin in top condition for its critical role.

There are several methods to get rid of toxins through the skin. We will discuss three of them: skin brushing, sauna and steam baths and detoxification baths.

Skin Brushing

This removes the outer dead layers of the skin and keeps the pores open. Toweling off vigorously until the skin is slightly red after bathing has a similar benefit. For this purpose towels have to be changed regularly as they remove the toxins. Since our skin is made up mainly of fats, applying natural high quality fats and oils helps to keep our skin healthy. Two excellent natural oils are butter and olive oils. To complement effective skin detoxification, you need good nutrition too. The wrong foods will just put back any toxin that you remove.

Sauna and steam baths

These are good ways to remove toxins from the skin and regenerate its vigor as a detoxifying organ. The sauna is a good follow-up to dry skin brushing because it pushes toxins out through the skin. The main thing to remember is to limit the time spent in a sauna. Perspiration is beneficial but too much heat can dry the skin, accelerating the aging process.

Detoxification baths

It is essential to take daily baths using natural soaps. Learn to care for your skin using only natural oils and products. We also need to carefully consider the materials that we wear as they can have a tremendous effect on our health. Natural fiber is favored over synthetic fiber as the former can help eliminate toxins.

> You may also want to consider a filter for your shower as most of us will absorb more toxins from bathing or showering than from drinking tap water.

Needless to say, swimming in the ocean is a much better option than in a chlorinated swimming pool.

A refinement of skin cleansing is skin brushing in addition to the detoxification bath. This is simple and relaxing. Try the following: Use either 1/2 cup of baking soda, Epsom salt or sea salt. Soak for 15 to 20 minutes and then scrub the skin gently with soap or a natural fiber. The water will turn murky and dirty within minutes as the heavy metal toxins (aluminum and mercury) are excreted from the skin.

Detoxification baths should be done once a week. When good health is restored, maintain your skin with a detoxification bath once a month.

> Always remember even though chemicalized skin care products such as soaps and shampoos may be cheap, they do not cleanse the skin of toxins. Absorbed into our body, they in effect add more toxins to our system. Most people fail to recognize the ill effects because their liver is able to metabolize the toxins. Yet, there are people who experience tremendous improvement in their health when they switch to natural soaps and shampoos.

C. Colon Cleanse

Colon cleansing has been practiced for 4,000 years to achieve detoxification. Through this process, the large intestine or colon can be healed, rebuilt and finally restored to its natural size, normal shape and correct function. There is no better place than the bowel to begin ridding your body of toxins and contaminants which may cause cancer, colitis, digestive disorders, fatigue and obesity. Many people are not aware that the walls of the colon are encrusted with toxins and fecal material. This toxic waste material has often been attached to the bowel walls for years. It is laden with millions of bacteria, which encourage disease and wreak havoc.

As the toxins are eliminated, many conditions such as skin disorders, breathing difficulties, depression, chronic fatigue, nervousness, severe constipation and arthritis are reduced in severity. This provides great relief especially when augmented with health-giving dietary changes and other treatment modalities. Patients should drink more unsweetened herbal teas and lots of water.

There are two stages to the therapy. The first is the cleansing stage involving a thorough washing of the large intestine. A sterile tube is inserted into the rectum and filtered warm water, or another suitable solution, is gently infused into the bowel. It washes around the colon. An evacuation tube removes the water which is allowed to travel all the way up to the cecum. Any encrustation is loosened, dislodged and flushed away. This goes on for about 15 minutes. The procedure is repeated at intervals.

The next stage is healing, rebuilding and ultimately restoring to maximum efficiency the colon's healthy function for the final absorption of nutrients and the total and timely elimination of all remaining digestive waste materials.

During the healing stage, a special infusion is introduced into the bowel that will cool inflamed areas and strengthen weak sections of the colon wall. Some of the common agents used in this stage include flaxseed tea, extracts of white oak bark and slippery elm bark. These herbs soothe, lubricate and introduce powerful healing agents directly into the large intestine.

Most people think of colon irrigation or enemas as an uncomfortable experience. It is, in fact, a very quick and effective way to wash away encrusted toxins. But if the thought of an enema bothers you, consider a colon cleansing diet instead. The plan is as follows:

Start with a diet of 50 percent raw food along with a teaspoonful of linseed or two level teaspoonfuls of Metamucil. Such bulking agents are readily available at pharmacies or grocery stores. Alternatively, you can chew linseed to release its beneficial nutrients. Water is an essential element in the cleansing process. Start the day with at least half a pint of water, preferably warm, before breakfast. Aim for two quarts per day while you are cleansing the colon unless this conflicts with the advice from your doctor.

D. Lung Cleanse

Aerobics exercise is widely associated with cardiovascular health. The less appreciated fact is that it also helps cleanse the lungs. During active and intense exercise, the force for exhaling is greatly increased to make space for fresh air. This forces out the dead air normally trapped within the small air sacs (alveoli) at the bottom of the lungs. The stale air with its load of gaseous waste from the lungs is expelled in exchange for oxygen-rich air. By this alone, it is important to exercise in non-polluted areas. When exercising for health, the last thing you want are pollutants from bad air.

Breathing exercises combined with physical activity coincidentally increase the action of lymphatic cleansing. This can be improved when you synchronize your breathing with the movement of your legs and arms. For example, when you are walking or jumping on the trampoline, inhale in four short draws and exhale in four short bursts. Move your arms and legs each time you take a small breath. Inhale through your nose and exhale through your nose or mouth.

E. Lymphatic Cleanse

When food is consumed, it is broken down and nutrients are sent to every living cell in your body. When the cells finish processing these nutrients, some waste is created. This waste, also called metabolites, must be removed from the body or it will "drown" in its own waste. The lymph system, which extends throughout the body, is the "highway" by which these wastes are transported from the cells to the blood, and then to the colon and kidneys for elimination. It is the sewage system of the body. In addition, it returns excess interstitial fluid to the blood, aids in the absorption of fats and fat-soluble vitamins from the digestive system, and transports these substances to the venous circulation. Furthermore, it acts as a defense against invading microorganisms and disease. Lymph nodes and other lymphatic organs filter the lymph to remove microorganisms and other foreign particles. Lymphatic organs contain lymphocytes, cells that destroy invading organisms.

When this system malfunctions or is blocked, toxic waste builds up and is kept inside the body, headaches, brain fog, memory impairment, fluid retention, chronic fatigue, muscle pain, eczema, fibrocystic disease, loss of energy, cancer, and frequent infections are just some of the symptoms of lymphatic system dysfunction and cancer.

An effective way of promoting circulation and flow of the lymphatic system is light massaging of the lymphatic channels and pathways that are located under the skin.

F. Kidney and Blood Cleanse

There is a good regimen for cleansing the kidneys. Like the skin, the kidney performs the task of continuously filtering out unwanted wastes and toxins from our blood to be expelled with our urine. To optimize this renal function, all we need is clean water to flush the kidneys out.

The rule is to drink one quart of pure filtered water daily for every 50 pounds of body weight. It is one of the absolute basic anti-aging fundamentals. If you are in good health, try drinking 10 to15 glasses of water daily. It is best to limit your intake to filtered or bottled water. The right kind of water is especially important. Distilled water is devoid of dissolved minerals and is, thus, able to actively absorb and eliminate toxic substances from the body. This is the basis for drinking distilled water during detoxification for a limited period of time (less than four weeks).

Once detoxification is accomplished, distilled water should be replaced with pure filtered water. Long-term use of distilled water can cause rapid loss of beneficial sodium, potassium, chloride and trace minerals leading to complications of mineral deficiencies.

Furthermore, distilled water can potentially over-acidify the body. When exposed to air, distilled water absorbs atmospheric carbon dioxide and becomes acidic with a pH of 5.8. The ideal water for long-term consumption should be neutral or slightly alkaline and contain minerals such as calcium and magnesium.

Water filtered through reverse osmosis tend to be neutral. When filtered through a solid charcoal filter, it becomes slightly alkaline. Both are recommended for daily drinking. Make sure that the filter you choose is of good quality. The best ones remove pollutants and parasites such as cryptosporidium. If you do not possess a water filter, bottled water is the next best option. It should however, be highlighted that about 25 to 30 percent of the bottled water sold in the United States comes from the tap— sometimes untreated!

G. Toxic Metal Cleanse

One of our most urgent needs in detoxification is to rid our body of toxic metals such as lead, arsenic, iron, cadmium, aluminum and mercury. These toxins disrupt normal enzymatic processes and so prevent the body from functioning properly and repairing itself. Premature aging and the development of disease is a sign of metal toxicity.

One of the best ways to cleanse the body of toxic metals is through chelation therapy. During the chelation process a synthetic amino acid called ethylenediaminetetraacetic acid (EDTA) is administered to the patient by a slow intravenous drip painlessly over three hours. Once in the bloodstream, EDTA works through a complex cascade of chemical reactions resulting in the binding of all the unwanted metals. These metals are then excreted through the urine.

As a result of the removal of toxic metals and calcium from atherosclerotic plaques, the vascular circulation system is improved through chelation therapy. For this reason, the therapy is one of the alternative treatments for patients with occlusive vascular diseases. Generally, oral chelation is not recommended due to the poor absorption of EDTA from the gastrointestinal track.

On the other hand, Mother Nature has provided us with some natural compounds that have chelating properties as well. The most important are:

Chlorella

Algae and other aquatic plants, such as chlorella, possess the capacity to take up toxic metals from their environment. Chlorella has been shown to develop resistance to cadmium-contaminated waters by synthesizing metal-binding proteins to mop up the dissolved metal. The complex carbohydrate in chlorella's cell wall, called mucopolysaccharides, absorbs large amounts of toxic metals rather like an ion exchange resin filter. It also extracts mercury trapped in tissues in the gut wall, muscles, ligaments, connective tissue and bone. In short, chlorella is one of Nature's more effective agents for toxic metal elimination, especially mercury and aluminum.

Using large doses of chlorella facilitates the excretion of mercury through feces. After the intestinal mercury burden is lowered, mercury will more readily migrate into the intestines from the other body tissues. Here chlorella will again effectively remove it.

Chlorella is not well tolerated by about one in three people due to the gastrointestinal distress it causes. Dosages vary from person to person and it is best to scale up slowly.

We will revisit the properties and powers of chlorella when we look at cancer-fighting protocols.

N-acetyl-cysteine

N-acetyl-cysteine (NAC) is another good natural chelator of mercury (possibly from dental amalgam fillings), cadmium and lead (for example, from paints and cigarette smoke). Because it is produced in living organisms from the amino acid cysteine, it is a natural sulfur-containing compound and a naturally powerful antioxidant as well. Having these dual properties make NAC both an indispensable nutrient in liver fortification and a tool in detoxification, currently.

NAC taken orally gets metabolized. It is also oxidized into an insoluble oxidate that may form kidney stones. As a preventive measure, vitamin C is taken to resist the oxidation.

3. Rebuilding

Now that you have gotten rid of the toxins in your body, keeping your body clean and toxin-free is very important. A rebuilding detoxification diet must provide us with nutritional fortification for restoring the body's immune system. A diet comprised mainly of fresh and simply prepared food is the best option for providing the necessary raw materials. Include raw green and colorful vegetables for fiber, vitamins and powerful micronutrients and antioxidants. The diet should be very low in trans- or hydrogenated fats, sugar, dairy products, caffeine, tobacco or other stimulants. Instead, drink plenty of water. Meats should only be consumed in small amounts and should be hormone-free. Rotate the food groups every four days to allow efficient digestion and excretion.

Starting on a clean slate, reinforce the body on a day-to-day basis. The following dietary adjustments are highly recommended.

Herbal Teas

The infusion of herbs in hot water has been drunk as tea through the ages. You can benefit from the wisdom gathered by the ancients and conveniently enjoy health-giving teas throughout the day. Herbal ingredients commonly used to enhance intestinal motility include: senna leaf, peppermint leaf, stevia leaf, buckthorn bark, damiana leaf, chamomile flower and uva ursi leaf. After the evening meal is a good time for enjoying some tea. Stevia leaf has to be taken with care as excessive amounts can cause abdominal cramps. Build up the habit slowly. Begin by steeping the tea just for one minute, in one to two cups of water, for the first three to five days. As your system adjusts, you may increase steeping up to five minutes. Most individuals will experience increased bowel movement or slight cramping during the first few days. This is due to the initial cleansing of the body's system and is normal.

Ideally, stool should be soft, smooth and easy to pass, but not watery. A good digestive enzyme taken with meals will normally result in this consistency. The herbal tea may cause it to be watery especially during the initial cleansing process. This is not uncommon. It should be noted that the consistency of stool varies greatly with each person. Adjust the amount of tea you drink to achieve the desired result. Suffice to say that watery motion should not be tolerated over time. It can lead to dehydration and electrolyte imbalance if ignored for too long. It is always a good habit to drink more water than normal during a detoxification and cleansing state.

Here is an example of a simple herbal cleansing program that can be used in conjunction with a detoxification diet.

- On rising: Drink a glass of lemon juice or plain water with an additional teaspoon of apple cider vinegar and a teaspoon of blackstrap molasses.

- Mid-morning: Drink a glass of plain water with added psyllium husk powder (which contains Metamucil) and another glass of water following that.

- With meals: Have two to three multi-digestive enzymes and liver herbs.

- Between meals: Drink herbal teas to support the liver.

Flora Supplementation

Optimal gastrointestinal health depends on the balance between billions of beneficial and pathogenic or disease-causing bacteria and fungi. Collectively they are known as our intestinal flora. The bad bacteria cause us no harm as long as the good ones are keeping them under control. A well maintained balance between these opposing microorganisms is essential for a properly functioning digestive tract.

About 400 species of these good bugs inhabit the intestines. Their total population is about 100 times the number of cells in your body. Remarkably, these microorganisms coexist peacefully in the carefully balanced internal ecosystem of our digestive tract. As long as they flourish, they prevent pathogenic bacteria and fungi from proliferating and causing trouble for us. The potentially pathogenic flora in our gut consists of *clostridia, salmonella, staphylococcus, Blastocystis* and *Candida.*

Research has shown that good bacteria, otherwise known as probiotics, help defend our bodies from bad bacteria and detoxify toxic chemicals. Their action produces valuable vitamins including biotin, folic acid, niacin, pantothenic acid, riboflavin, thiamin, vitamin B6, vitamin B12 and vitamin K.

The bacteria assist in our digestion of proteins and fats, too. Lactose intolerance caused by our inability to digest milk properly can be cured with probiotics. Good bacteria also ensure that toxins are excreted from the bowels rather than absorbed into the bloodstream. They even improve the stool texture and the time it takes to clear the bowel. Amazingly, improving our intestinal floral balance relieves dermatitis as well.

One such good bacterium is acidophilus. They stimulate activity in the thymus and spleen, both key immune system glands. They prompt our body to manufacture natural antibodies. Certain acidophilus strains even protect against the formation of tumors and promote production of interferon, a hormone that protects against cancer.

Replacing our natural flora is vital to keeping our bowels healthily populated with good bacteria. In particular, Lactobacillus acidophilus and Bifidus can help us in our detoxification program.

Acidophilus supplements are widely available in health food stores and drugstores. Selecting from among the numerous "what-have-you-dophilus" products may appear a daunting task. Examine the labels and you will discover a variety of useful bugs including Lactobacillus acidophilus, Bifidobacterium bifidum, Lactobacillus bulgaricus and Streptococcus faecium. Some products may contain fructo-oligosaccharides, which are sugars that nourish beneficial bacteria to make them colonize faster. All of these ingredients are acceptable and any combination of them works well.

Remember that acidophilus supplements contain living organisms, so freshness is critical. Purchase a product well before its expiration date, which should be clearly stated. Once the cartons are opened, keep them refrigerated. Discard any remainder that is more than six months old. Dosage varies from one product to another. It is best to refer to the instructions on the label.

If you do not wish to consume supplements, try yogurt, which contains the friendly bacterium Lactobacillus acidophilus, a well established probiotic.

Enzyme Supplementation

Digestive enzymes are chemicals that speed up or catalyze certain reactions in the body. In fact, there are over 1,300 different types of them. These enzymes are the "chemists" who facilitate the extraction of all our bodily raw materials. They break down our food into substances to be absorbed by our alimentary canal and are very specific in their action. For example, the enzyme lipase only acts to break down fats. As we recall, vitamins A, D, E and K are fat soluble. They can be obtained from the fatty meats that we consume provided that we can break down the fat to release the crucial vitamins. This illustrates how important enzymes are.

However, cooking and processing food can destroy enzymes. Without the digestive catalyst, the delivery of nutrients to our system is affected. On top of that, toxins from undigested food will accumulate in the body. We consume an average of two pounds of food per day or 20 tons over a lifetime. A smooth passage of food through the gastrointestinal tract is critical to avoid stasis of feces and its release of toxins.

Fortunately, plant enzymes have properties similar to ours and can act as substitutes. Raw fruits and vegetables contain a plentiful supply of enzymes. Supplemental enzymes have also proven to be helpful. So before you go and spend a fortune on vitamin pills, check to see if your problem is a lack of enzymes not releasing the vitamins into the body's system.

On an interesting note, one of the early signs of benefit from supplementing digestive enzymes is an improvement in skin tone. Undernourished skin quickly loses its glow. Restoring its nourishment will immediately be apparent. In addition to consuming raw food and mineral supplements, supplementation with digestive enzymes is clearly an important part of anti-aging treatment.

Green Whole Food Supplement with Key Nutrients

This list of whole food supplements incorporates many of the nutrients that were first mentioned when we discussed the liver's detoxification pathways.

A. Amaranth

Amaranth is one of America's oldest crops. It was first grown in Central America in 2000 B.C. and reached its zenith during the Aztec civilization. During his reign, Emperor Montezuma stored tons of amaranth for five to ten years to withstand the ravages of drought, famine and pestilence.

A high proportion of it is protein (including lysine and methionine), calcium, iron, potassium and phosphorus, as well as vitamins A and C. Amaranth also contains tocotrienols (a form of vitamin E). It also contains about 6 to 10 percent of unsaturated oils. It is concentrated in linoleic acid, which is important in human nutrition.

B. Spirulina

The Aztecs were also first to discover this wonderful and amazing herb that looks like blue-green algae. Found in abundance in Lake Texcoco in Central America, it was the main source of protein, principally gamma-linolenic acid (GLA), in their daily diet. Besides mothers' milk, no other known source provides as much GLA. Spirulina contains 25 times more carotene than carrots and six times more protein than eggs. It has an extraordinarily high digestibility coefficient of 95 percent.

In other words, 95 percent of the proteins, enzymes and living essences are absorbed into our bloodstream very quickly without loss of energy.

Spirulina is a biogenic food. This means that it is a living, enzyme-rich raw food that has its own unique abilities to promote great health. Like chlorella, it has strong chelating powers to absorb unwanted toxic heavy metals and also some forms of xenoestrogenic toxins from our body.

You will read more of other "green" foods like spirulina in a later section on fighting cancer.

C. Flax

Another ancient herb, flax is a soluble fiber that has been grown in the Mediterranean for over 5,000 years. Flax can be crushed and used as a mild and safe laxative. It comprises 20 percent of omega-3 fatty acid which is useful for reducing serum cholesterol.

> **Together with lignans, the omega-3 fatty acid helps to reduce blood glucose. This omega-3 component provides an excellent source of nutrient to enhance the liver detoxification pathways. Flax also contains other proteins and all the essential amino acids for maintaining total wellness. Flaxseed oil is a good alternative if flaxseed is not available.**

However, this oil has a tendency to turn rancid rather quickly and takes second place when compared to fish oil as a source of omega-3 fatty acid. It is recommended that you choose flaxseed grown in a cold country such as Canada.

D. Millet

The discovery of millet as an exceptional nutritional source had an unexpected beginning. During World War I, with famine staring them in the face, millions of Russians were forced to eat the millet that they had stored for their chickens. It was very pathetic for them, resorting to eating animal feed. But much to everyone's surprise, no one died of starvation. After the war, Dr. Kellogg studied the grain and discovered that it had a better balance of vitamins and minerals than wheat, barley, oats, rice, or rye.

Millet actually contains incredible amounts of iron, B vitamins and potassium. It is also a very affordable solution for weight watchers as it is low in calories and oils. Millet contains the right amount of fiber and can be digested easily. It also has exceptionally low allergy rates.

E. Chicory

This old but most complete herb was first cultivated in Egypt. Its fields were irrigated by the flooding of the Nile 5,000 years ago. The ancient Egyptians believed that the herb could purify the blood and the liver and used it as medicine. Research studies have shown that two of the substances in chicory, namely lactucin and lactucopicrin, can counteract the stimulant effects of caffeine by their sedative action on the central nervous system. Herbalists consider chicory a mild tonic, diuretic and laxative. Taking chicory on a regular basis can help to lower cholesterol levels. Due to its bitter taste, which somewhat resembles that of coffee, it is often used as a healthier substitute.

Summary

The concept of detoxification as a way to hormonal balance and reduction of estrogen cannot be overemphasized. Our body has an internal detoxification system in place. In the case of hormonal balance, no other organ is more important than the liver. Unfortunately, our liver is overloaded with junk food and toxic chemicals, and often not functioning at its optimal state of clearing excess estrogen from the body. This contributes to estrogen dominance. No estrogen reduction program can be completely successful without detoxifying the body. It is simply not possible. Fortunately, there are natural compounds and modalities that can help, many of which have been explored in this chapter.

Chapter 9

Your Diet

Maintaining Ideal Body Weight

Obesity is fast becoming a worldwide problem. We have established that the connection between obesity and estrogen is very strong. The minefield of estrogen-related illnesses has been described in some detail in Chapter 5.

The standard index for base-lining obesity is the body mass index or BMI, which is calculated by dividing your body weight in kilograms by the square of your height in meters. BMI of between 18.5 and 25 is considered healthy. Those with a score between 25 and 29 are classified as overweight. BMI higher than that is considered obese. Ideally, the target weight should be five to ten percent below one's body weight.

Your ideal body weight can be calculated easily. For women, the formula is 100 pounds plus five pounds for every inch above five feet. Therefore, for a woman standing five feet six inches tall, the ideal weight is 100 + (5 pounds per inch x 6 inches) = 130 pounds, give or take five pounds for a large or small frame person respectively.

Half of the adults in Europe and 61 percent of American adults are overweight. Obesity is so prevalent that it is considered epidemic in some communities. The implications in medical costs, at the national and personal levels, are of grave concern.

If you are overweight, it would be advisable to shed as much of your fat tissues as possible. Do this with medical advice as too sudden a reduction could hurt your health or would not be sustainable at any rate.

Dietary Adjustments

Over-eating and under-exercising are the norm in developed countries today.

Populations from such countries, especially in the Western hemisphere, derive a large part of their dietary calorie from fat. Sadly, in large urban communities, obesity seems to be prevalent among the poor. They also show a much higher incidence of menopausal symptoms brought on by estrogen dominance. It is time to eradicate the problems with proper education about nutrition.

A good solution is dietary adjustment. Studies support the switch from a typical high-fat, refined-carbohydrate diet to a low-fat, high-fiber, plant-based diet. Such a switch effectively brings down the estrogen level. Plants give us many vitamins, minerals, and enzymes. They contain 5,000 known sterols that have progestrogenic effects.

Communities used to eating more wholesome food and who exercise more have a far lower incidence of menopausal symptoms.

This solution would not be complete without removing the social habits that would undo all the good derived from the new diet. We need to wean ourselves of caffeine, alcohol, tobacco and other such toxins that are so commonly consumed.

Adopting a healthy eating lifestyle and diet is, however, easier said than done. It is uphill all the way. But the sense of well-being and achievement at the end of the hard climb cannot be bought.

1. Cruciferous Vegetables

Scientists have found the so-called cruciferous vegetables such as broccoli, cauliflower, cabbage, kale, bok choy, watercress, broccoli and Brussels sprouts to contain a high level of phyto-estrogens. These important vegetable estrogens compete to occupy the estrogen receptor sites on the cell membrane and prevent a woman's excess estrogen from exerting its full effects on the cell. About three to five servings a week are needed to reap this benefit.

Consumption of these vegetables can be helpful to those suffering from estrogen deficiency or very early stages of estrogen dominance. Avoid over-consumption of phytoestrogens which, in excess, can give rise to estrogen-caused ill effects. After all, plant estrogens are estrogenic in nature. It is not recommended for those afflicted with fibroids, fibrocystic breast disease, or cancer to take cruciferous vegetables.

Many cruciferous vegetables also contain a compound called indole-3-carbinol (I3C) which is part of our detoxification supplement regime. This compound has been shown to reduce the risk of hormone-dependent cancers such as prostate, breast and ovarian cancer.

2. Liquids

The body needs water to perform many functions. Digestion and elimination of bodily wastes cannot proceed without it. For everyday consumption nothing beats safely filtered water. This simple drink has fallen out of favor as people get ever more sophisticated and adventurous. We now discuss the ills that arise from the social drinks that we consume.

Coffee

A body of evidence shows that drinking more than two cups of coffee a day may increase estrogen levels in women. We have quoted earlier the clinical study showing that women who consumed at least 500 mg of caffeine daily, the equivalent of four or five cups of coffee, had nearly 70 percent more estrogen than women who consumed less than 100 mg of caffeine daily.

There is now wide acceptance of the fact that caffeine intake from all sources is associated with higher estrogen levels regardless of the woman's age, body mass index (BMI), or other attributes. On this evidence alone, it is best for women with endometriosis, breast pain and a family history of cancer, to start turning off coffee.

More than that, coffee also creates an acidic internal environment especially when sweetened with sugar. The body, in trying to neutralize the acid, will withdraw valuable minerals such as magnesium and calcium from the bone. Such mineral depletion, if unchecked, will contribute to osteoporosis.

As a stimulant, caffeine gets the adrenal glands pumping. For a woman with estrogen dominance this speeds up adrenal fatigue.

Alcohol

Avoid alcohol or drugs that tax the liver, the premier detoxification center in the body. The overtaxed organ will lose its efficiency. For those with hormonal imbalance it will lead to an increase in estrogen. The metabolism of estrogen slows down in an alcohol-damaged liver as it slowly loses its metabolic efficiency on estrogen.

Water

Water, filtered through reverse osmosis or a charcoal filter, makes the best staple drink. Ideally, it should be neutral in pH or slight alkaline. While distilled water is pure, it has the tendency to remove minerals from our bones. It is also advisable to avoid fluoridated water and all chemically treated tap water. Tap water contains varying amounts of chlorine from country to country. While chlorine is an effective treatment against microorganisms, it also has detrimental effects on human health.

> **It is perhaps sensible to invest in a water filter for the home. We should also bathe or shower in filtered water. We repeat the warning that bottled water can sometimes come straight from the tap. This is true even in America.**

3. Organic Food

An earlier chapter laid out the economic reasons that drive the majority of farmers to depend on pesticides and herbicides in their farming methods. When ingested, these toxic compounds mimic the hormone estrogen and upset our hormonal balance. There is today a worldwide trend away from produce dosed with pesticides and other chemicals.

Choosing only organic food will help us avoid diseases caused by xenoestrogens like breast cancer. Pesticide and herbicide-free organic foods also contain higher quantities of vitamins and minerals than foods grown in commercially fertilized and toxin-laden soil.

Similarly, farmers often inject hormones and antibiotics into their livestock in order to hasten their growth and keep them alive until they go to market. The farmers claim that these drugs are stopped weeks before market. Yet there is evidence that much of the xenobiotics are retained in the fat tissues for months. For your own health buy organic eggs, meat and dairy products whenever you can and keep away from the rest. Look for the organic food label from a reputable organization.

4. Soy

In the last ten years, soy has gone from an obscure food to the perfect nutrient. Promoters of soy products would like you to believe that soy is the healthiest food you can eat. They base their claim on soy's extensive history in the Asian diet and the long lifespan of Asians as a group.

However, a closer examination will show that the Asian diet is not focused on soy at all. In fact, 65 percent of the calories in the typical Japanese diet comes from fish. In China, 65 percent of calories come from pork instead. The total caloric intake from soy in the Chinese diet is only 1.5 percent. The amount of soy consumed in Asia averages only two teaspoons a day and up to a quarter cup in some parts of Japan. In contrast, new converts to the soy fad are wolfing down soy products. Their intake can be as much as eight ounces (220 grams) in a serving of tofu steak and two glasses of soy milk.

Another consideration is the way soy is consumed in Asia— typically it is first allowed to ferment from six months to three years. Only then is it eaten—and as a condiment, not as a meat substitute. Fermented soy includes miso, tempeh and natto. Natto, a pungent fermented soybean paste, has been enjoyed in Japan for over 1,000 years. It is rich in vitamin K2, a critical nutrient for bone building. It also has the extraordinary property of dissolving blood clots and keeping our blood vessels clear.

> In sharp contrast, unfermented soy such as soymilk is the second most common allergen in the world. Studies have shown that 30 grams of unfermented soy consumed daily can affect thyroid function and is strongly linked to a host of auto-immune diseases such as Hashimoto's thyroiditis as well as hypothyroidism. Its antagonism to the thyroid hormone is well established.

Eating unfermented soy in a strictly vegetarian diet actually increases the risk of mineral deficiency including calcium, magnesium, copper, and zinc and the consequent vitamin D deficiency. This is due to the antinutrients present in soy. For example, fresh soy contains phylates, an antinutrient which blocks the body's absorption of minerals from the gastrointestinal tract. It also contains enzymes inhibitors that reduce protein digestion.

Other studies have shown that women observing a high soy diet had a higher incidence of changes in their body's cellular structure consistent with malignancies such as epithelial hyperplasia.

The evidence against soy seems to be mixed, however. Some evidence even suggests that processed soy protein contains carcinogens such as nitrates and lysinoalanine. Other studies have shown that taking 35 to 60 gram a day of soy protein, containing aromatase inhibitor genistein, can protect the body against breast cancer.

However, it is advised that soy be avoided for anyone wishing to reduce her body's estrogen, especially those with concurrent thyroid problems.

Summary

Maintaining your ideal body weight is best done with a diet high in raw vegetables, hormone-free meat, if meat is taken, and low in unfermented soy. On the other hand, avoid eating excess cruciferous vegetables which contain phytoestrogens that aggravate estrogen dominance. All these are primary parameters in an estrogen reduction diet.

Chapter 10

Lifestyle

We now look at an aspect of the health risks that we have control over. It is the way we live, the lifestyle we choose. This is something we grow up with and, as easy as it sounds, it will take a lot of self-discipline and strength of conviction to change. Some changes are easier than others, but all of them lead you to better health and vitality.

1. Exercise

Properly performed, exercise has been shown to modulate hormonal imbalance through the menopausal years and beyond. Those who exercise regularly are also happier, less depressed, and have an optimistic outlook on life. This results in an increased life expectancy. Statistically, life expectancy increases by two hours for every hour spent doing proper exercises.

In a study of 1,550 women between ages 40 to 85, both with and without breast cancer, it was found that those who started exercise early in life had the greatest reduction in cancer risk. The risk reduction was as much as 50 percent for those who have consistently exercised for 20 years. This is after adjusting for factors such as smoking history and weight. In a comprehensive review by Dr. Marilie Gammon and her colleagues at the Columbia University School of Public Health, 11 out of 16 investigations on recreational exercise reported a decrease in risk among both premenopausal and postmenopausal women between 12 and 60 percent. The study was published in the *Journal of the National Cancer Institute* (Jan 21, 1998).

In one of the largest studies, where 25,000 women were tracked for 20 years in Norway, it was shown that women who exercised at least four hours per week, during leisure time, reduced their risk of breast cancer by about 37 percent. Even jobs that entailed high levels of activity, such as lifting and walking, reduced breast-cancer risk by 25percent. Exercise has also been found to be helpful to breast-cancer survivors as well as those who have undergone some breast-cancer treatment.

Just how does physical activity resist the development of breast cancer? A combination of factors may be at play. Knowing now that obesity adversely affects our hormonal health we have a few clues. People who exercise tend to be thinner. Steroids normally stored in fat are turned into estrogen when fat tissues accumulate. These all spell estrogen dominance in clear print. The longer the woman's system is exposed to an excess of estrogen, the higher her risk of developing cancer.

Exercise also moderates the adrenaline caused by stressful lifestyles. We have read how adrenal exhaustion can lead to diabetes. As an added bonus, exercise can give your heart a real boost as well. Studies have shown that even light exercise benefits heart health, although longer and harder regimes are better.

A complete exercise routine must incorporate flexibility, cardiovascular and strength training. All it takes is five minutes of flexibility training every day, 20 to 30 minutes cardiovascular training three times a week, and 15 to 20 minutes of strength training twice a week. A properly structured program takes an average of 30 minutes a day—less than two percent of the entire day.

Given the fact that 75 percent of pre-metastatic cancer cases occur in postmenopausal women, it is imperative that all women, especially those after menopause, embark on a program of regular and moderate physical activity. The sad reality is that seven in ten adults do not regularly exercise and nearly four in ten have a totally sedentary lifestyle. It appears that warnings about physical inactivity have been ignored. There has been no notable change in the lifestyle statistics in the West [my addition] from 1997 to 2001.

2. Xenoestrogens Avoidance

The scientific community took up the challenge of determining how the modern urban environment so adversely affects women's health. It was all the more intriguing that women in rural communities showed few of the symptoms seen in their sisters in the city. Over the last few decades, with technological advances in their research, scientists have demonstrated that certain synthetic chemicals are to blame.

These chemical compounds we have identified as *xenoestrogens*. They disrupt the normal hormonal processes in men, but especially in women. In the body, they react with endocrine glands that secrete hormones, including the sex hormone estrogen. By mimicking estrogen, they confuse the system that controls the estrogen released. So our next advice is to keep away from these counterfeit hormones.

The problem is that xenoestrogens are used in a variety of products that most people come into contact with all the time. Many of the common detergents, wetting agents and preservatives used in popular-brand cosmetics, household cleaning products and so forth, contain chemical substances that are estrogenic to our human body. In 1988, the FDA reported that 30 percent of cosmetic products on the market contained these substances.

Bearing that in mind, here are some tips to heed:

A. Plastics

Try to limit the use of plastic goods since all plastics leach chemicals into our environment. Many households are fond of using plastic containers and plastic wrap to store their food. These materials often contain plasticizers, which give them their flexibility. Plasticizers are potential xenoestrogens. They can easily migrate into the food especially during reheating or cooking in a microwave oven. To lessen the harmful effects, choose polyethylene if you have to use plastics. It does not have the same deleterious properties. A better alternative is to use glassware for such purposes.

B. Pesticides and Herbicides

Avoid pesticides and herbicides such as DDT, endosulfan, dieldrin, methoxychlor, kepone, toxaphene, chlordane and other chlorinated hydrocarbons. There is conclusive evidence that they are xenoestrogens. Exercise caution when selecting your food. Opt for organically grown produce. Apart from your vegetables, lawns and golf courses may also be tended with a generous dose of estrogen-like pesticides and herbicides. Some of these, for example, DDT, are known carcinogens, too. They can easily enter our bodies through skin contact and our lungs.

C. Phthalates

Phthalates are xenoestrogenic plasticizers used to make vinyl. More than that, vast quantities of phthalates are also used in many leading beauty care products that you may be using everyday, including hair spray, deodorant, antiperspirants, hair gel, nail polish, nail polish remover, and perfume.

Phthalates have been shown to damage the lungs, liver, and kidneys. They have also been known to degrade sperm, causing infertility. The solution is to use organic, phthalate-free cosmetics products.

D. Ortho-phenylphenol Products

Ortho-phenylphenol is a chemical widely used in disinfectants. It took some time but now both the Environmental Protection Agency (EPA) and IARC have classified it as carcinogenic. This substance may be present in Lysol Disinfectant Spray, which is widely used in hospitals, clinics and homes. You are advised to use other non-toxic disinfectants instead. Try using vinegar and water as household cleaner.

E. Bleached Products

Many of our common household products like coffee filters, paper, napkins, toilet tissue and tampons have been bleached for esthetic effect. However, the EPA has filed an alarming report stating that using bleached coffee filters can result in a lifetime exposure to dioxin, another xenoestrogen, beyond the acceptable level of risk. Clearly the best advice is avoid bleached materials. There are chlorine-free products in the market. Ask for paper products whitened without chlorine. Hydrogen peroxide is the safer bleaching agent.

It is also more environmentally friendly. Many factories' waste products, including chlorine, are dumped into rivers and other water sources.

3. Sleep and Melatonin

We all know that sleep is absolutely important to our wellness, but few appreciate that sleep deprivation can kill us! Sleep research is gathering momentum and it is revealing some startling facts about the true value of sleep. Our energy, efficiency, clarity of mind, and ultimately our mental attitude depend, to great extent, on getting enough good quality sleep. Much of the benefit of sleep comes from generating enough melatonin, a hormone produced in the pineal gland. Secretion of the hormone is increased when we are sleeping in total darkness. Quite apart from the other benefits of sleep, there is a direct relationship between estrogen, estrogen receptors and the ability of melatonin to inhibit cancer growth. It is explained by the fact that a high melatonin level is positively correlated with an increased progesterone output, which in turn corrects estrogen dominance. Sleeping 8 to 10 hours a night in a completely dark room to increase melatonin production is the key. Try going to sleep before 10 p.m. Sleeping early is also important due to the adrenal-restorative and cortiso-hormone balancing effect. One hour of sleep before midnight has the health-beneficial effect equivalent to two hours of sleep after midnight in this respect.

4. Clothing

Recall that the lymphatic system is partly responsible for transporting nutrients, immune agents, pathogens, and toxins in the maintenance of our body's health. What happens when it is restricted? This is especially so for women who wear overly-tight under-wire bras, training bras or girdles.

Scientific studies have reported that the chance of getting breast cancer increases with the length of time spent in a tight brassiere. The constriction from tight clothing chokes lymphatic drainage. Pools of unhealthy toxins and pathogens eventually cause damage to tissue cells. To the extent that is socially acceptable, dispense with the bra. Wear clothing as loose fitting as possible so as not to cut off the lymphatic drainage system.

5. Preservatives

Many toiletries contain dangerous preservatives that may give you cancer. Whether it is a shower cream or even baby bath soap, you could be absorbing these carcinogenic chemicals into your body each time you wash your hair, take a bath or even bathe your baby. These preservatives include methyl paraben, ethyl paraben, propyl paraben and butyl paraben. The toxic chemicals are absorbed via our skin into the bloodstream. We have already noted that absorption is ten times more efficient via the skin compared to our gut.

Again the solution is to use organic lotions and shampoos.

6. Hair dyes

One can only speculate that people who dye their hair are ignorant of the cancer risk they are taking. The fact is as many as 20 percent of all cases of non-Hodgkin's lymphoma are directly linked to regular use of hair dye. Even though the FDA has not required a warning label for hair dyes, their toxicity has been verified by several studies. Grecian Formula, for example, contains lead acetate, which damages the nervous, circulatory and reproductive systems when it is absorbed through the skin.

Vegetable-based dyes, without those synthetic ingredients, are the safer alternative.

7. Miscellaneous Strategies

Xenoestrogens are found in many other everyday items in any average home and office. New carpets and fiber boards emit vapors from solvents; photocopiers and printers give off some noxious fumes, gels in diaphragms and condoms use unsafe lubricant surfactants, and X-rays and computers generate dangerous electromagnetic fields. All of these cause a lot of damage to our body chemistry in the long run. Avoid them if there is a choice.

Summary

To reduce estrogen load, avoid commercial plastic and choose glassware instead for containers. Similarly, avoid chemical-laced beauty and household products like the plague. Substitute with organic household and beauty care products. They may be more expensive but the price is worth paying when you weigh up the savings you realize in peace of mind, if not hard medical costs.

Chapter 11

Jane's Story—A Message Of Hope

Now that we have understood the principles behind keeping our hormones balanced, let us review the story that we began with—Jane's sorry history. With our grounding in this subject, we can now begin to play medical detective and say what went wrong and how it could have been different.

First, Jane's history, as far as her hormones are concerned:

1. Taking birth control pills at age 16–that was the in thing to do—was a wrong decision, especially given her family history of breast cancer.

2. She started neglecting her physical exercise and did not curb her liking for sweets. Unnoticed, overweight crept up on her. Estrogen is made in the fat cells.

3. Taking on the responsibilities of a homemaker after marrying, she exposed herself to many xenoestrogens in the environment of a modern home. Xenoestrogens behave like estrogen once inside our body.

4. She assumed a high-stress position at work and kept at it for long hours and long years. Chronic stress compromises the adrenal glands, leading to reduction in progesterone and an increased level of estrogen.

5. Like everyone else, she drank more coffee than was good for her. Caffeine stimulates estrogen. Even when she decided to cut it down, she switched to tea which

did not prove much better since tea is a good source of caffeine.

6. Her work obliged her to entertain and partake of a diet too rich in meat and alcohol. Meats are often laced with estrogenic hormones, while alcohol reduces liver function, leading to an increased estrogen in the body.

7. Quite unknown to her, the street lamp that shone into her bedroom, lessened the melatonin her body could put out. The lack of the hormone sapped her energy and sense of well-being.

8. Then she developed PMS and should have gone for a total hormonal workup but instead bravely ignored the warning signs.

9. Since PMS has its root in estrogen dominance, she should have taken immediate steps to cut down her sugar, increase her physical activity, rein in her weight, reduce her workload and taken natural nutritional supplements that counter the excess estrogen.

10. When she was told of her uterine fibroid at age 42, immediate steps should have been taken to further reduce her exposure to xenoestrogens. She also should have then started on bio-identical progesterone to offset her own excess estrogen.

11. When she had the total hysterectomy at age 48, she should have insisted on an androgen workup and possible androgen replacement as well. Furthermore, she should have refused estrogen-only hormone replacement therapy.

12. Finally, her doctors should have raised the alarm over her risks because of a family history of breast cancer.

As it turned out, she was ignorant of the danger signs. She was a "sitting duck," a breast-cancer time-bomb waiting to go off. What Jane suffered, millions around the world are going through every day still. It is by no means unique to her alone. Her story is a classic, one I have encountered over and over again in my practice. Yet each body is different. Some people are blessed with a stronger genetic disposition and are able to avoid developing breast cancer. But the odds are against you if you do not take heed and eliminate estrogen dominance. You may be running on borrowed time.

Unfortunately, nothing can be done to rescue the past. Jane's uterus and ovaries are gone; her cells have been flooded in estrogen over 30 years of neglect and her breast-cancer cells are out of control. That is the reality Jane has to deal with now.

But let us for one moment suppose that she awakened in time to the fact that there are good alternative approaches to treating her condition. What if after extensive investigation and talking with numerous experts in natural medicine, she decided to find a natural solution?

Say she goes for a total checkup without wasting any more time. She then realizes that her estrogen load is the root cause of her woes. It is likely that she has a thorough hormonal workup. She learns that natural progesterone can reduce the problem. The mainstream recommendations will be tempered with her newly-acquired knowledge of how natural products augment the treatment. She is seriously taking responsibility for her own health ...

What Are Jane's Options, Knowing What We Know?

Knowing what we know now, Jane decides to keep her options open. The following is a possible different route through her history.

First of all, she decides against radical breast surgery (mastectomy). Instead, Jane opts for natural therapies. Pursuing a course of intensive detoxification and a hormone reduction program, using the wide variety of nutritional and other mechanisms we have detailed above, will prepare her to fight the disease more effectively. This means going for a series of scans to track the cancer growth. Her doctors will simultaneously check if her cancer markers are reduced. If the tumor shrinks, she will not need surgery. It will be enough to continue her natural therapy.

Even if her cancer is not arrested, Jane will be physically better prepared to face the surgery. Her body and immunity will be strengthened by the natural nutrients. Her antioxidants will make the cancer more susceptible to chemo- and radiotherapy.

Reducing Estrogen Level

Jane finds a doctor who is oriented towards natural therapies, one who has a background in orthomolecular oncology (that is, who fights cancer with high doses of natural nutrients). The doctor helps her design a natural cancer treatment program to run concurrently with her treatment by a regular oncologist. Her orthomolecular program will be tailored for her weight, age and physical condition.

1. Natural progesterone cream is prescribed to balance her estrogen. She also avoids taking food with a high concentration of phytoestrogens such as broccoli to avoid their estrogenic effect.

2. She begins a modified diet that includes whole foods, vegetable juices and low-glycemic fruits. Her sugar intake is kept to a minimum and filtered water is her only choice of fluid. No tea, no coffee. She is allowed only plant not animal proteins. She avoids cruciferous vegetables and unfermented soy products such as tofu.

3. She works on reducing her weight without sacrificing nutrition. This also helps her to reduce estrogen secretion from her fat tissues.

4. She avoids the use of plastic containers by switching to glass. Commercial shampoo and beauty products are replaced by organic based products.

5. She begins an aggressive nutritional supplementation program to help clear as much estrogen out of her body as possible, using a variety of natural compounds including methionine, NAC, milk thistle, vitamin C, vitamin E, folic acid, magnesium, chromium, innositol, choline, quercetin, taurine, GABA, calcium d-glucarate and alpha lipoic acid.

Fortifying the Defenses

Next Jane aids her body in combating her cancer by getting rid of the toxins that have weakened her defenses. She goes through a fast and practices skin cleansing to flush the toxins out. Alternatively, she embarks on a modified Gerson Detoxification Program. Vegetable juicing and herbal teas rebuild her liver's function. She follows a diet low in hormones and high in raw vegetables.

Meanwhile, the addition of fish oil, digestive enzymes, flaxseed and probiotics in her new diet restore her gastrointestinal terrain as well as its pH balance. The cocktail of nutrients—plant proteins, complex starches, essential fatty acids, minerals, vitamins, enzymes, antioxidants and plenty of water—in her diet are absorbed with gusto into her system. She gets all the nutrients her body needs for the good fight.

Lastly, having regained her strength, she increases her level of physical exercises. Her adrenal and thyroid glands are rejuvenated. The relief this regimen brings to her stressful life is further enhanced with a stress-reduction program and psychotherapy if there are underlying causes.

Initially the lifestyle change is very difficult for Jane. She suffers from slight caffeine withdrawal symptoms. The whole food taste needs getting used to. But with great determination and will power, she excels in the program.

After intensive detoxification, hormone rebalancing and immunity-building for the first four weeks, she is feeling great. It has not been easy, but she is determined to beat the cancer and prevent its recurrence. As her body realigns with nature, she gradually finds that toxic foods (such as French fries) actually turn her off. She continues her nutritional supplements and with the help of her doctor, she adjusts her dosage every few months to match her dynamic condition.

At the same time, she also goes for regular scans and diagnostic tests to ensure that all is well. As long as her scans show no new cancerous mass, Jane is comfortable to continue her program of natural therapy. She has avoided surgery and chemotherapy and is rebuilding her body's immune system and rebalancing her hormones to fight the cancer.

The natural treatment for Jane's cancer has been hugely successful. Nevertheless, she does not rule out conventional therapy and her regular oncologist is kept abreast each step along the way. She will go for it if it becomes necessary. Until then, she is beating cancer naturally.

Jane's strong fighting spirit proves to be a critical factor in her recovery. She has undergone a remarkable transformation in her lifestyle. Her positive outlook has been crucial in conquering her breast cancer.

The moral of the story is quite simply: Look before you leap. There are alternative treatments for breast cancer.

Epilogue

Modern society has brought with it many external hormonal insults to our body. Such insults manifest themselves in symptoms associated with menopause, PMS and premenopausal symptoms. It is apparent that the common thread among these symptoms is relative estrogen dominance. Today experts are telling us that the majority of the symptoms and syndromes can be prevented and reversed if early steps are taken to reduce the estrogen load. The vast majority of these symptoms can be avoided by lifestyle adjustments alone.

In absolute terms, all of us living in a developed world are soaking in a sea of estrogen. The food we eat is often laced with xenoestrogens: The air we breathe; the shampoos we use; the plastics around us; the birth control pill or hormone replacement therapy, all exacerbate estrogen dominance.

For the professional, working life is stressful. It leads to adrenal exhaustion and hormonal complications, if left unchecked. The lifestyle habits we choose add toxins to our system and take away the physical activity that our body sorely needs. We delay childbearing and restrict the number of children we bear. It increases the average woman's lifetime exposure to estrogen in her bloodstream.

Then there are well-intentioned doctors who have not kept in touch with the leaps in advancement in the science of ortho-molecular oncology. They believe that the symptoms suffered by such patients are part of life and leave the problem to fester. They often prescribe unopposed estrogen supplements without knowing the full story and add to the estrogen torrent. When the cancer comes to a head, they recommend the only treatments they know: surgery, chemotherapy and/or radiotherapy. Frequently these drastic and traumatic approaches are unnecessary if the patient's fundamental problem of hormonal imbalance is solved.

In principle the solution is simple. In practice it requires much strength of conviction to make fundamental changes in a lifestyle that we have grown accustomed to. But with the right frame of mind it can be done. The reward is a quality of life—pain-free, zestful and happy—that many have forgotten.

About the Authors

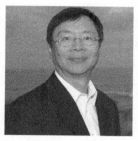 **Michael Lam, M.D., M.P.H., A.B.A.A.M.,** is a western trained physician specializing in nutritional and anti-aging medicine. Dr. Lam received his Bachelor of Science degree from Oregon State University, and his Doctor of Medicine degree from the Loma Linda University School of Medicine in California. He also holds a Master's degree in Public Health. He is board certified by the American Board of Anti-Aging Medicine where he has also served as a board examiner.

Dr. Lam is a pioneer in using nontoxic, natural compounds to promote the healing of many age-related degenerative conditions. He utilizes optimum blends of nutritional supplementation that manipulate food, vitamins, natural hormones, herbs, enzymes, and minerals into specific protocols to rejuvenate cellular function.

Dr. Lam was first to coin the term, *ovarian-adrenal-thyroid (OAT)* hormone axis, and to describe its imbalances. Dr. Lam was also the first healthcare professional to scientifically tie in Adrenal Fatigue Syndrome (AFS) as part of the overall neuroendocrine stress response continuum of the body. He systematized the clinical significance and coined the various phases of Adrenal Exhaustion. He has written four books: *The Five Proven Secrets to Longevity, Beating Cancer with Natural Medicine, How to Stay Young and Live Longer, and Estrogen Dominance.*

In 2001, Dr. Lam established *www.DrLam.com* as a free, educational website on evidence-based alternative medicine for the public and for health professionals. It featured the world's most comprehensive library on AFS. Provided free as a public service, he has answered countless questions through the website on alternative health and AFS. His personal, telephone-based nutritional coaching services have enabled many around the world to regain control of their health using natural therapies.

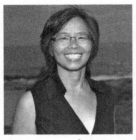 **Dorine Lam, R.D., M.S., M.P.H.,** is a registered dietitian and holistic clinical nutritionist specializing in Adrenal Fatigue Syndrome and natural hormonal balancing. She received her Bachelor of Science degree in Dietetics, holds a Master's Degree in Public Health in Nutrition, and a Master of Science degree in Nutrition from Loma Linda University, in Loma Linda, California. She is also a board-certified, Anti-Aging Health Practitioner by the American Academy of Anti-Aging Medicine. She coauthored with Michael Lam, M.D., the book *Estrogen Dominance* and numerous articles on Adrenal Fatigue Syndrome. Her personal research and writing focuses on the metabolic aspect of Adrenal Fatigue Syndrome.

She is married to Michael Lam and is an integral part of the telephone-based nutritional coaching team helping people overcome Adrenal Fatigue Syndrome.

Made in United States
North Haven, CT
28 February 2022

16593508R00119